TAME YOUR APPETITE

THE ART OF MINDFUL EATING

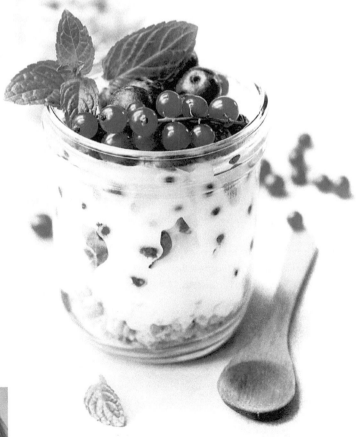

SHEILA H. FORMAN, PH.D.

TAME Your Appetite: The Art of Mindful Eating

Published by TVGuestpert Publishing

Copyright © 2022 by Sheila H. Forman, Ph.D.

ISBN-13: 978-1-7358981-2-4
BISAC CODES: HEA006000, HEA017000, HEA010000

Nationwide Distribution through Ingram & New Leaf Distributing Company.
This publication is designed to provide accurate and authoritative information in regard to the subject matter covered. It is sold with the understanding that the publisher is not engaged in rendering legal, accounting, or other professional service. If legal advice or other expert assistance is required, the services of a competent professional person should be sought. – From a Declaration of Principles Jointly Adopted by a Committee of the American Bar Association and a Committee of Publishers and Associations.
Some names and identifying details have been changed to protect the privacy of individuals. All brand names and product names used in this book are trademarks, registered trademarks or trade-names of their respective holders.
TVGuestpert Publishing is not associated with any product or vendor in this book.
TVGuestpert Publishing and the TVG logo are trademarks of TVGuestpert, Inc.
TVGuestpert & TVGuestpert Publishing are subsidiaries of TVGuestpert, Inc.
TVGuestpert & TVGuestpert Publishing are visionary media companies that seek to educate, enlighten, and entertain the masses with the highest level of integrity. Our full-service production company, publishing house, management, and media development firm promise to engage you creatively and honor you and ourselves, as well as the community, in order to bring about fulfillment and abundance both personally and professionally.

Front Book Cover Design by Lynn Pelkey
Book Design by Carole Allen Design Studio
Author headshots by Cathryn Farnsworth
Edited by TVGuestpert Publishing

11664 National Blvd, #345
Los Angeles, CA. 90064
310-584-1504
www.TVGuestpertPublishing.com
www.TVGuestpert.com
First Printing 2022
        10 9 8 7 6 5 4 3 2 1

DISCLAIMER

The information, ideas and suggestions offered in this book are not intended as a substitute for professional advice. Before following any of the suggestions offered, you should confer with your medical and mental health professionals to make certain that the information is right for you. Neither the author nor the publisher shall be liable or responsible in any way for any loss or damage alleged to arise from the information contained herein.

In addition, throughout this book you will find "case studies." Each case study is a composite of various experiences presented for illustration purposes only. Any resemblance to any person, dead or alive, is merely a coincidence.

A word about weight loss—mindful eating is a non-diet approach to weight management. It is not a diet or quick weight-loss program. Some people lose weight with this approach; others do not. Some initially gain weight when they abandon previous restrictions. The research on mindful eating says that the more you practice mindful eating techniques, especially mindfulness meditation, the greater the likelihood for sustainable weight loss. Because weight loss depends upon your own efforts, body type, and medical and psychiatric history, the author and publisher make no guarantees regarding weight loss.

Lastly, although Dr. Sheila Forman is licensed to practice psychology in the State of California, no psychotherapist–client relationship has been established by the information presented in this book, nor by any program or product Dr. Forman has created.

◆ ◆ ◆

DEDICATION

    This book is dedicated to the mindfulness community of which I am proud to be a part. Thank you for bringing mindfulness to the world at a time when distractions and pain fill our lives. I believe that as mindfulness permeates the zeitgeist, joy and peace will fill our hearts.

    This book is also dedicated to the memory of my beloved mother and father who always believed in me and always believed I would succeed. Thank you, Mom and Dad. I miss you both every day.

◆ ◆ ◆

Do not blindly believe what others say. See for yourself what brings clarity and peace. That is the path for you to follow.

Buddha

ACKNOWLEDGMENTS

Hillary Clinton famously said that it takes a village to raise a child. Well, the village I have created for myself helped me create this book. Without these extraordinary people, this book would not have come into being.

I must start with Dr. Jean Kristeller and Andrea Lieberstein who provided the research and the training in Mindfulness-Based Eating Awareness (MB-EAT) which is the foundation of my *TAME Your Appetite* work. Thank you for your meaningful contribution to the field of mindful eating and your generous offering of training, mentoring, and support. It is my privilege to be able to assist in spreading the word about the benefits of MB-EAT and mindfulness in general. Without you, I wouldn't have gotten started on this path.

My next thank you goes to my MB-EAT colleagues: Dr. Helen Luna, Sara Solomon, Victoria Davis, Grace Hallinan, Carmen Popo, Patti Badiner, Karla Goplen, and Maria Rippo. You all added greatly to my learning the MB-EAT program and provided support and encouragement as I launched TAME. From teachbacks to Skype sessions to FaceTime and emails, you were all an important part of this journey for me. I hope you can see your contributions within these pages.

Next, I offer my heartfelt gratitude to my accountability partners: Dr. Gretchen Kubacky, Diane Curran, Judy Ludy, Karen Owoc, Linda Dennis, and Brian Dennis. Our weekly, monthly, and bi-monthly accountability sessions kept me on track and focused. Each interaction was a reminder of my purpose and intention. For that, I am very grateful.

This book got its start because of the remarkable mentoring of Jacquie Jordan and support of Stephanie Cobian. Jacquie, thank you for believing in me and this book from the moment I told you about it. You gave me the confidence that I was on the right track.

To my goal-setting partners, Madge Beletsky and Deirdre O'Conner, thank you for our goal-setting dinner dates and success stickers. Your constant encouragement for even the smallest successes moved me forward each and every month. I enjoy our mutual support and look forward to continuing it indefinitely.

Finally, I want to thank the clients who have welcomed me into their lives, shared with me their pain and frustrations, and whose remarkable changes have made me want to keep doing what I'm doing.

◆ ◆ ◆

×

TABLE OF CONTENTS

FOREWORD

You may have picked up this book because of your curiosity about mindfulness, or your desire to expand an existing mindfulness practice. Or perhaps you're seeking a lasting solution to a long struggle with food or your weight. Congratulations! You're about to find your way to a peaceful and lasting relationship with food, as well as with many other aspects of your life.

As a health psychologist specializing in chronic illnesses that often have a component of eating disordered behavior, such as binge eating, I am always looking for resources that will offer my clients new skills to improve their health. I am pleased to introduce Dr. Sheila Forman's excellent book on mindful eating and am already recommending her TAME program to my clients.

Dr. Sheila is your smart, savvy, and compassionate guide on this journey of self-discovery. She is an accomplished psychologist, author, speaker, and teacher. To this, I would add that she is a forward-thinking innovator in the field of mindfulness, especially as it relates to mindful eating. This book is the crystallization of her years of professional experience as a psychologist, teacher, and practitioner of mindful eating. She has interwoven the details of her own experience of acquiring the skills of mindful living and mindful eating, complete with frustrations and how she overcame them. She will ease you almost effortlessly into a new way of thinking, with easily implemented exercises designed to guide you into a state of equanimity around food.

Dr. Sheila has taken a complex subject and broken it into a practical, simple, and meaningful series of steps and practices. Each part of the practice is based on well-developed and tested theories that have been proven to produce calm, focus, and an improved relationship with food and your eating practices, behaviors, and beliefs. Should you still doubt the potential of mindful eating, she also supplies ample research to back up her assertions, as well as suggestions for further reading and practice.

Our family histories, culture, and social lives are all factors in our relationship with food, and may have contributed to stress, fear, anxiety, and unhealthy eating behaviors. Mindful eating will take the stress out of your food choices and bring peace to something that should be simple and easy.

Enjoy the process of reading and implementing the practices in this book. Observe how your body begins to relax, along with your mind. Know that you have already made a very good decision to read this book, and trust that you have the capacity to create meaningful and mindful changes in your relationship with food.

To your health!

Dr. Gretchen Kubacky
Health Psychologist and Author of,
The PCOS Mood Cure: Your Guide to Ending the Emotional Roller Coaster

◆ ◆ ◆

Introduction

The beginning is the most important part of the work.

Plato

Does this sound like you? You are unhappy with how much you weigh. Despite being smart, educated, and successful in other areas of your life, you find yourself overeating when you don't want to or know you shouldn't. You are frustrated because you keep regaining any weight you might lose.

You find yourself vowing to solve your weight problem by going on yet another diet, signing up with a personal trainer, or exercising it away. Or you are at a point in life when you are thinking life is too short, you'll never be at a weight you'd be happy with, so you might as well give up?

Stop! Before you sign up for another weight-loss program, fork over thousands of dollars at the gym, or shove a Snickers bar in your mouth, hear me out.

Your usual ways of trying to manage your weight haven't worked for you because the truth is diets are only temporary solutions, excess exercising can lead to injury, and neither of these options address the emotional and mindless aspects of eating.

The truth is, you are not alone, and, most important, you are not a failure. We live in a world where it is becoming harder and harder to maintain a healthy weight without a lot of effort. Our world's obesity epidemic is at an all-time high. People everywhere are struggling to lose weight and keep it off. And despite our best efforts and the newest diet plans and promises, we are failing miserably. Worse yet, with each additional diet, we are gaining more and more weight.

But don't worry. There is hope. I have a way out of your struggle with weight and your war with your body. I know. I've been there and I have used what I am about to share with you to release the excess weight that I was unhappy with and to make lifestyle changes that have led to peace with food and my body. I am no longer plagued with concerns about what to eat, when, or how much. I have learned to trust myself in such a way that I can distinguish between emotional and physical hunger and make choices that are ultimately in my best interest. I can truly say that I healed my relationship with food.

As a psychologist specializing in weight and eating issues, I have seen every diet and approach to weight management out there and am a leading expert in helping people end excess eating. I have studied what works and what doesn't work. Having had my own struggle with weight, I have even experimented on myself.

After twenty years as a psychologist helping people manage their weight by managing their emotions, I was frustrated by the lack of progress some of my clients were making trying to lose weight and keep it off. I found they had a hard time differentiating physical hunger and emotional hunger, identifying feelings of fullness, and coping with their emotions without turning to food. I knew that what they needed was a way to change their relationship with food. I also knew that what I needed for them was a different approach.

Always the student and always in search of information to help those I work with (as well as myself), I dove back into the research on food, eating habits, and weight management. In doing so, I came across the work of Dr. Jean Kristeller of Indiana State University and Mindfulness-Based Eating Awareness Training (MB-EAT). Dr. Kristeller is the pioneering researcher in the field of mindfulness-based eating and author of *The Joy of Half a Cookie.*

After reading her book, I researched some more and learned about Dr. Kristeller's professional training program. I enrolled in the program and began my journey, both professionally and personally, into mindfulness and mindful eating.

When I applied mindfulness and mindful eating to the work I was doing with my clients, I realized that these were the missing pieces to successful weight management and peace with food.

Mindful eating does not focus on weight loss but rather on becoming more aware of patterns of inappropriate eating and providing tools for making sustainable changes in these patterns. It is designed to increase mindful awareness of eating habits and decrease mindless and unhealthy ones.

Based on a foundation of daily mindfulness meditation and mindfulness-based tools and techniques, MB-EAT teaches a new way of relating to food and eating. It explains how to create balanced eating and experience true gastronomic delight and satisfaction. This leads to enjoying food more, eating less, and ending the cycle of deprivation, overeating, and guilt.

I discovered that mindfulness-based eating could be your path to weight loss and peace with food as you learn how to gradually shift away from your current eating habits into healthy mindful ones. With mindful eating, you will go from policing yourself to honoring yourself. From mindlessly reacting to food and emotions to mindfully responding instead.

In the pages that follow, I will reveal what it has taken me my lifetime to acquire. In this book, you will learn mindfulness-based eating awareness techniques which will allow you to lose weight, keep the weight off, and manage your emotions without the need for another diet or exercise plan.

I will teach you tools such as Mindfulness Meditation, Inner Wisdom, and Outer Guidance, and I will walk you through a precise step-by-step program to regain control over your eating, manage your emotions, lose weight, keep it off, and finally feel at peace with food.

Your journey into mindful eating will mark your goodbye to emotional, mindless, and binge eating; good-bye to yo-yo dieting; good-bye to excess weight; and good-bye to the battle between your appetite and your body. You will gain the skills necessary to eat according to your own body's needs, to address your emotions in healthful ways (such as using meditation) and to lose the extra weight you've been carrying around. As a bonus you will feel happier, healthier, and more relaxed.

Meet Allison. Allison was morbidly obese when her primary care physician suggested she try therapy as a way to lose weight. Reluctantly, Allison called for an appointment. She had been on many diets and really wasn't interested in going on another one. When I explained to her that I don't use diets to help people deal with their weight issues, she agreed to come in.

During our first session, I told Allison about mindful eating and how we will use meditation and other mindful techniques to get her eating under control. She rolled her eyes at the thought of meditation, telling me how she didn't think it would help, and that nothing did. But since her doctor had scared her so much with talk of health complications from diabetes and even perhaps an early death, she agreed to give it a try.

I took her through a short breathing meditation (like the one I will teach you in Step One) and then sent her home with two simple instructions. First, do ten minutes of meditation most days. Second, pay attention when she eats. There were no rules or guidelines as to what she should or could eat, only to pay attention. Concerned that she might have wasted yet another hour on a useless approach, Allison agreed to give it a chance. We scheduled our next session for the following week. When Allison returned, she was smiling. She began talking about her week before we even got settled into our seats. She started by telling me how she left the previous session sure that what I suggested was useless but, after talking it over with her husband, realized she had nothing to lose and followed through.

Allison shared a lot with me during that session but what she said about the subtle change in her eating habits without even trying was most important. She told me that by simply paying attention to what she was eating, she naturally ate less.

She reported what I hear over and over again. By paying attention, she noticed she was eating foods that didn't really taste good to her, so she ate less of them. She also noticed that when she paid attention, she recognized fullness sooner than when she was distracted and, consequently, was able to leave food on her plate. Bingo! She got it!

As for the meditation, Allison said that while she struggled to stay focused on her breath, she appreciated the ten minutes of solitude. Works for me! I was very pleased. Allison was on her way to becoming a mindful eater and a healthier person.

As Allison learned, when you eat mindfully and pay attention to your food, you will choose quality over quantity and satisfaction over rules. Allison grasped how by simply paying attention when she eats, she will regain control over her eating and lose her excess weight. Allison was optimistic and excited about what the future would hold for her.

I would like that optimism for you, too. Won't you join me in this new approach to an old problem? An approach that uses both 21st-century science and age-old wisdom. An approach that uses mindfulness and mindful eating instead of food plans and treadmills.

Using the approach outlined in this book you will establish a meditation practice, become acquainted with your own innate wisdom on which foods nurture your body best, learn how to balance eating with nutrition and health information without resorting to another diet, explore your emotions without overeating, and discover how to use mindfulness as a tool to enhance your entire life, not just your eating habits.

All you'll need to get started is a willingness to pay attention. Here's what you will learn:

In Chapter One, we will expand our conversation about the current state of the obesity epidemic and the prevalence of mindless eating. We will look at how the food, diet, and advertising industries have set us up for weight management failure. Do we really need ten different types of cream cheese or prepackaged noodles that can be cooked in a cup? You will see the extent to which mindless eating and emotional overeating have infiltrated our lives and the negative consequences that follow. Who hasn't regretted eating a pint of ice cream after being "good" all day? Or lost a weekend to a food binge instead of being with friends and family? You will be shown how, by letting go of a diet mentality, you can come to trust yourself to decide what foods and amounts are right for you and how you can use mindfulness as a tool for dealing with your emotions without having to turn to food to cope.

In Chapter Two, I will take you through my journey of how mindfulness and mindful eating helped me deal with my excess weight and how I then used what I learned to help my clients. This chapter will highlight my personal struggles and success with weight management and eliminating emotional eating (i.e., from using food to cope as I pursued my first career as an attorney to dealing with the hormonal ups and downs of menopause and how I got past all that), as well as, other success examples. This chapter will also introduce you to mindfulness in general and how you can start incorporating mindfulness into your life right away—no fancy Zen retreat or a trip to Nepal necessary. The chapter will conclude with an explanation of how mindfulness will benefit your health and overall well-being.

In Chapter Three, you will be shown my five-step mindful eating plan which is based on the *TAME Your Appetite: The Art of Mindful Eating* workshops and coaching programs. In doing so, I am giving you an opportunity to utilize this powerful program on your own. You will do the famous "Raisin Exercise" as your entry into mindful eating. If you are worried that you can't do this, I address the obstacles to getting started and how to overcome them. Because of the information in this chapter, you will no longer feel obligated to "Eat! Eat! Eat!" even as your mother (husband, friend, lover…) pushes food in your direction. Because of this chapter, you will know what to expect and how to set yourself up for success.

In Chapter Four, I teach you the first step to mindful eating—mindfulness meditation. I will explain the value of meditation and how it is essential to mindful eating, and I will also give you instructions on how to meditate, meditation script included. You will get information regarding a suggested practice schedule, keeping a meditation log, and the use of meditation tools (i.e., cushions, benches, timers, etc.), as well as tips on what to do when problems arise, such as when a kitten wants to join the meditation practice, or a cell phone keeps beeping across the room. Through this chapter, I will hold your hand to help you get comfortable establishing a practice.

Next, in Chapter Five, I take you through the second step of mindful eating—cultivating Inner Wisdom. I will explain what Inner Wisdom is and why it works better than a diet or other outside recommendations. We will explore the elements of Inner Wisdom—hunger, thirst, fullness, taste, satiety, and satisfaction—individually, and each discussion will include an exercise and a meditation. For example, in the Mindful Taste section of this chapter, I will guide you through an exercise using brownies. Yummy.

In Chapter Six, I introduce you to Step Three—the importance of using essential nutritional and health information to inform mindful eating choices. The information is called Outer Guidance and is used to help you decide what, where, when, and how much to eat. I'll explain the difference between Outer Guidance and "going on a diet." I will also give you examples of Outer Guidance (i.e., calories, portion sizes, nutritional information, product labels, organic vs. natural food products, clean eating, Weight Watchers, etc.), as well as how to gather Outer Guidance (i.e., book, blogs, webinars, etc.). Furthermore, I will offer my own successful experience of identifying and employing Outer Guidance. By the end of this chapter, you will feel confident to trust your own instincts to determine what Outer Guidance serves your needs best.

Chapter Seven explains Step Four. In this chapter, I will show you how to experience your emotions without using food as a crutch. If you have been caught in a cycle of "emotional eating-dieting-bingeing-emotional eating," this Step can really make a difference. As you will learn, the key to this Step is the question: *What are you really hungry for?* In answering this question, you will learn to identify your emotions (anger, anxiety, boredom, sadness, loneliness, hopelessness, and stress) and what you can do besides eat when you feel those emotions. Again, meditation will be taught as a foundation. I will show you other mindfulness-based tools which you can use, including mindful writing. In case you discover that you are in need of deeper work, I will show you how to get extra help.

Chapter Eight concludes the five-step plan. Step Five will show you how using mindfulness can enhance other areas of your life. The benefits of mindfulness meditation on your health (i.e., decreased stress, anxiety, depression, pain, and insomnia) are explained. Exercising mindfully will be introduced, as will mindful cooking. I will show you how approaching all of life in a mindful way (i.e., while washing dishes or doing chores around the house) can be a way to increase your wellness and overall happiness. I'll also give you tips on getting better at mindfulness, such as how you can practice being mindful while sitting at a traffic light or on hold with the cable company. In time, you will find that the more you practice mindfulness, the easier it becomes and the more benefits you will enjoy, including changes in your weight. Being mindful is not hard, it just takes practice.

Chapter Nine pulls together all the elements of mindful eating with a retreat. Since not everyone has the time, resources, or interest to attend a fancy retreat, and since you don't need an expensive or lengthy one to enjoy its benefits, I will show you how you can have a retreat right at home. I will use my own experience with daylong and silent retreats to give you recommendations on how to create a retreat for yourself. Of course, if you are interested in attending a retreat, I will offer suggestions on how to pick a suitable one for you. To facilitate your stay-at-home retreat, I will provide preparation instructions and a recommended schedule.

Suggestions for How to Use This Book

If you are brand new to the idea of mindful eating, or if you have never meditated before, I would recommend starting from the beginning and working your way through the steps in the order they are presented. The steps truly are steps and flow naturally from one to the next. They are consistent with the original Mindfulness-Based Eating Awareness Training (MB-EAT) research that is the basis for this program, and thus build a strong foundation that can serve you well.

I would also recommend that you spend at least one week on each step. More might even be better. You are developing a new set of skills and there is no need to rush. It is very likely that in learning these steps you will be undoing a lifetime's worth of poor habits. Habits that are entrenched will take time to replace. So go slow. Savor each step. Move on when you feel as if you've "got it!"

On the other hand, if you feel stuck, frustrated, or are on the verge of giving up, move on anyway. You can always come back to the step that stymied you. Remember you cannot do this process wrong. As you will learn, mindfulness is about "beginning again." Jammed up by a step? No worries. You can always come back to it and "begin again" when the time is right for you. What is important is that you continue through the steps in a compassionate, non-judgmental, and patient way. Our goal is consistent, not perfect, practice. Be kind to yourself.

If you are familiar with mindful eating or have an established meditation practice, feel free to begin wherever you are. At some point, I think it would be valuable for you to visit all five steps, but if you are eager to add to what you already know, dive in at whatever step feels right for you. Be flexible. Move back and forth through the material in whatever way feels right to you. Again, we are emphasizing consistency, not perfection.

Before we move on, I want to tell you: you can do this! Mindful eating has, as a core element, being in touch with your body, with your "self." You started out in life in touch with your "self." As a baby, you knew very well when you were hungry, thirsty, or tired. You still do. It's still in there. It just may be covered up with decades of thoughts, habits, and experiences that created a disconnect. This five-step program will help you reconnect with yourself in ways you simply don't remember. As you will see, you will gain so much more than peace with food when you embrace these five steps.

One more suggestion. If you are open to it, I suggest you start a journal to record this journey. As you will learn, writing can be an excellent mindful skill. Before you get to that though, I believe that keeping a journal can help you see where you've been, and when and how you might be stuck. Use a journal in whatever ways work best for you—daily, weekly, as needed, in the morning to start your day, or at night before you go to bed. Writing down your food is not part of the five-step program but doing so can help to see how your eating habits change over time. Just be sure to use your food record as a tool for information and not as a way to restrict your food intake.

Are you ready to change your relationship to food and become a mindful eater? Good. Let's begin.

◆◆◆

Chapter One
Mindless Munching and Emotional Overeating

The best predictor of future behavior is past behavior.

Mark Twain

TOO MUCH OF A "GOOD" THING

As a nation, we eat too much food. The typical American eats 1,996 pounds of food every year. That's almost a ton of food per person, averaging about five pounds a day. Wow, that's a lot of cheeseburgers! So why do we do this? Why do we, intelligent, law-abiding, rational people, eat so much?

I have come up with several reasons:
- The ubiquitous nature of food in our society;
- The machinations of the advertising industry which set us up for weight loss failure; and
- The mindlessness that permeates our relationship with food.

Let's look at each reason more closely and see how each affects your attempts to manage your weight. First, the omnipresence of food in our world.

FOOD AT YOUR FINGERTIPS

Wherever we go, we are given the opportunity to buy food. It used to be that food was available only in grocery stores, candy stores, and restaurants. Slowly but surely, food has become available to buy everywhere. Think about it. Gas stations used to sell gas and oil. Today, gas stations have mini-marts attached to them offering corn dogs, oversized drinks, and nachos. Drugstores used to sell medications, cosmetics, and other personal care items. Now they have aisles filled with canisters of chips, packages of nuts, and two-pound bags of caramel-filled chocolates. Stationery stores sold office supplies. Now office supplies include tubs of licorice, buckets of popcorn, and cases of soft drinks. You may even find human candy and snacks available for sale in pet stores. Be careful though, some of the pet treats look like people food! But that's a topic for another book. Even Starbucks, which started out selling only coffee, now offers food for every meal.

Certainly, having food available at various locations can make running errands a bit easier since you don't have to make as many stops. But having food so readily obtainable makes us vulnerable to overeating in general and to making poor food selections specifically.

Much of the food that is so easy to grab-and-go tends to be highly processed, chemically ladened food which, while tasting awesome, is not good for any of us. I challenge you to find the nutritional value of a sprinkled donut or a king-sized nugget bar. Yet we eat these foods, and others like them, literally by the tons. Eating these foods might fill us up, but they don't nourish us, making us a country of overfed yet malnourished people. You don't have to be a poverty-stricken child in a remote village to be malnourished. Your body can be "starving" in a wealthy industrialized country like America because it is deprived of vital nutrients not found in heavily processed foods. If you ever wonder why you get so many colds, feel low in energy, or have high cholesterol, just look inside your shopping cart.

Also, being constantly presented with so many food options challenges our decision-making ability, leading us to make poor choices. Research tells us that we have a limited capacity for making decisions and that with each decision we make, we exhaust that reserve. Scientists call this "decision fatigue." Decision fatigue means that the more decisions you make during the day, the harder your brain must work. Urban legend has it that the reason Facebook CEO Mark Zuckerberg always wears the same type of clothing is that "it is one less thing to think about." I can imagine how that would be a good thing for the owner of a major company like Facebook.

You might not run a billion-dollar company, but you do make hundreds of decisions every day about what to wear, where to park, whom to call, which email to answer and what to eat. It can be exhausting. When it comes to making good food choices, an understanding of decision fatigue and how it wears us down and weakens us is important. When we are suffering from decision fatigue, it takes too much effort to think through food choices, making it easier to impulsively pick pizza over salad for dinner.

Choices based on impulse are common. Choices made impulsively, meaning without conscious thought or consideration, often reflect habit and can be called mindless decisions. On the other hand, choices made with attention and forethought are more likely to be mindful decisions, which are the kind of decisions that will serve your weight loss goals well.

Before learning to be mindful, most of us make choices out of impulse or habit. For example, you see a chocolate chip muffin that looks and smells really good, so you reach for it and take a bite without considering whether you are hungry or if this muffin is what your body needs at this moment. Biting into the muffin reflects an impulsive, mindless decision. But what if you looked at the muffin, considered whether you are hungry, and assessed if this muffin would taste good to you now? Whatever choice you make—to eat or not eat the muffin—now reflects a more mindful decision.

Keep in mind that decisions made earlier in the day when we are fresh and energetic are more likely to be mindful, healthy ones than those made later in the day when we are tired and worn out. It becomes easier to overeat, especially unhealthy foods, as the day goes on. Over time, this can have significant consequences for our health and our weight.

Our food environment is not the only reason why we eat too much. Some of the blame lays with advertisers and how they get into our heads.

MADISON AVENUE IN YOUR BRAIN

We live in a world where you can't watch TV, read a magazine, or even do a Google search without being bombarded by advertising. I remember when cable television first came into being. Sure, you paid a monthly fee for access, but you didn't have to endure commercials. That's not true anymore, is it? I miss those good old days of uninterrupted time with my favorite shows. That was real binge-watching! Instead, today, our television shows are filled with advertisements for everything from cars to vacations to fast food. And it is not just TV.

We are blasted with ads everywhere. Go to the gas station to fill up your car and there is a screen playing ads. The same is true for doctor offices, airports, and on the radio in our cars. These ads encourage us to eat all sorts of food and connect doing so with joy, love, happiness, and success. Eat a cheeseburger and a beautiful woman will wash your car. Share a bag of nacho chips and you're the coolest kid in town. Toast some waffles and your children will definitely eat breakfast with you. On and on it goes.

Truth be told, we want those things the commercials reflect, and advertisers know that. They use our desires to sell their products by creating a strong association in our minds between their products and those desires. This is not marketing voodoo; it is scientific fact. If you ever studied psychology, you might have heard of Ivan Pavlov and his famous dog experiments where he taught his dogs to salivate to the sound of a bell. Out of his experiments came a term known as "classical conditioning." Classical conditioning refers to a learning process that occurs when two items or events are paired together and become associated. In the matter of Pavlov's dogs, he paired meat with a bell. The dogs would salivate when they smelled the meat and eventually learned to salivate when they heard the bell even though no meat was present.

Advertisements work on the same premise. Companies spend a lot of time and money to condition you into pairing their products with particular events, feelings, and behaviors. You want a happy family, make a one-skillet dish for dinner tonight. If you are stressed, reach for a candy bar for relief. You want a romantic evening, be sure there are strawberries and chocolate nearby. You want to lose weight, drink milk. These are examples of some of the associations that we come to believe to be true because of advertising. And it's these associations that lead to mindlessness and mindless eating.

Scientists from institutions such as Yale University and the University of Liverpool are actively engaged in research proving that food ads make us eat more. Without conscious effort, we are at the mercy of these savvy marketers. The good news is that with mindfulness you will be able to interrupt these messages with a message of your own. I'll explain more on how that will work later on.

For now, let's dive a bit deeper into the mindlessness pool by looking at what role mindless and emotional eating play in our dilemma.

MINDLESS AND EMOTIONAL EATING

As an introduction to this topic, answer the following few questions. If you see yourself in them, that's okay. That's why you are here.

A FEW QUICK QUESTIONS:

1 Do you eat without paying attention, often reaching the bottom of a bag or bowl and wondering how you got there?

2 Do you always order the same food when you go to a familiar restaurant, regardless of whether you might prefer something different that time?

3 Is it your habit to visit the snack bar whenever you go to the movies or sporting event?

4 Is one of the first things you do when you get home opening the fridge door?

5 How about when you are visiting your parent(s) or grandparent(s)? Do you reach for the fridge then, too?

6 At the end of the day, do your reward yourself with something delicious, feeling like you earned it?

7 Is your initial response to an uncomfortable feeling to eat something?

8 Do you eat when you are lonely? Angry? Sad?

9 Do you look forward to the weekends so you can "let loose" and eat whatever you want?

10 Does eating junk food leave you feeling bad about yourself?

If you answered yes to any (or all) of the above questions, you do, or have, eaten mindlessly and/or emotionally. But no worries. You are in the right place.

The truth is we are all mindless and emotional eaters from time to time.

These behaviors have infiltrated our lives, causing negative consequences, physically and emotionally. If you lean towards the dramatic, you might say that mindless and emotional eating are threats to our well-being.

Years ago, when families gathered around the dinner table after a hard day's work in the field or at the shop, mealtime was special. Attention was paid to the food served. Gratitude was expressed for those who prepared the meal. The day's events were replayed, and topics of the time were discussed. The purpose of the meal was for the family to eat together as a unit. Nothing else mattered. Nothing else was going on. Today, this kind of family dinner is virtually nonexistent. Parents and kids eat at different times and often different foods. Today, we eat on the run. We eat while we drive. We eat while doing other things like watching TV, texting on our cells, or working on the computer. In a word, today we eat mindlessly.

Mindless Eating is eating without paying attention to what you are doing. It is not noticing quantity or quality. When we eat mindlessly, we eat without regard to our body's needs. We don't know if we are hungry or thirsty. Fullness and satiety don't register. Neither does taste satisfaction. All of this can lead to excess food and often the wrong kinds of food. It is the exact opposite of mindful eating.

Occasional mindless eating in and of itself is not terrible. Mindless eating becomes a problem when it is your habitual form of eating. When you consistently eat without regard to your body's needs, you risk damaging your health, diminishing your energy levels, and putting on extra weight.

Emotional Eating can do the same. Emotional Eating is eating in an effort to deal with feelings. For example, you just had a frustrating conversation with a superior at work. You are so angry you can barely contain yourself. The next thing you know you are standing in the break room in front of a box of donuts. You grab one and bite into it. You take another bite and then a third. You are starting to feel better. You can feel your body relaxing. The temporary boost in your serotonin and dopamine levels from eating that sugary, highly processed donut shifts your mood. Suddenly you are not as mad as you were moments ago. You grab another donut and head back to your desk. By the time you get there, the rage you felt at your superior has faded and you go back to work. That's emotional eating.

The problem with emotional eating is that it is a short-term solution. The boost in your serotonin or dopamine levels might lift your spirits, but that lift is brief. While you might be feeling better, the problem that caused the emotional distress remains, and now you have consumed extra food that your body wasn't hungry for, which can lead to excess weight and damage to your self-esteem.

If that isn't bad enough, our struggles with weight aren't due to just our eating too much. We are also guilty of eating the wrong foods. But don't feel bad. It's not your fault.

IS THAT FOOD?

When was the last time you ate a Twinkie? Those creamed-filled cakes were childhood staples for me. There was always a box in the cupboard, alongside Chips Ahoy! cookies and Rice-A-Roni. Sadly, these childhood memories are examples of what I now call the "wrong foods," highly processed food-like substances which cause disease, act addictively within our bodies, and leave us malnourished. They might look like food, but they are not.

Have you ever taken a moment to look at the label of a typical box of processed foods or tried to read the label aloud? The words listed are hard to pronounce, aren't they? Even if you can pronounce them, do you know what they are? Here, try one: sorbitan tristearate. This chemical is a stabilizer used in food and aerosol sprays. I found it in the ingredient list on a box of cookies. Here's another: tricalcium phosphate. This chemical is a type of salt known also as bone phosphate lime. It is used in many products—toothpaste, baby powder and antacids. This ingredient was on a popsicle box. What is it doing in our foods?

These hard-to-pronounce words are not foods at all. They are manufactured substances used to enhance flavor, increase shelf-life and, as some researchers theorize, cause us to want to eat more (to become addicted). By making processed foods more appealing, these "non-food" ingredients lead us to make unhealthy choices. We reach for these foods when we are hungry, thinking that we are eating food. We are certainly consuming calories. But as far as our body is concerned, it's still hungry. Why? Because these highly processed foods are full of nasty ingredients that do not nourish us. Apple juice made from water and concentrate is not the same thing as a crisp ripe apple. Frozen yogurt filled with artificial flavors and coloring is not the same as a cup of whole Greek yogurt and fresh berries. Your body knows the difference. It is looking for the nutrients that will restore, repair, and nourish it.

If you find yourself wanting more food after eating what should have been a full meal or snack, it is very likely the cause of your desire for more food is your body's search for nutrition. Because of this search, you end up eating more food and gaining more weight. When you can feed your body "properly" and give it what it needs, you will naturally eat less, and your weight will move in the direction it needs to go. So, how do you do that? Simple. With mindful eating.

AND NOW FOR SOMETHING DIFFERENT

If you have been trying to get rid of excess weight the traditional way, you have probably gone on a diet. You have probably gone on many diets. What the diet industry doesn't want you to know, and what science is proving, is that diets don't work. Diet schemes demanding low calories damage metabolism. Those that rule out one or more food groups create imbalance. Others skimp on vital nutrients. Most, regardless of their approach, are unsustainable. The truth is, if any of them worked, you wouldn't be looking for something new.

For me, the most compelling reason why diets don't work is that diets take us away from our true selves. Diets disconnect us from who we really are and require that we listen to some authority outside ourselves. Diets impose upon us rules and recommendations that might or might not be right for our particular body. You might follow a diet which tells you to eat animal protein at every meal or snack. That suggestion may be appropriate for some people but not for you because it makes you sluggish. Or another diet might tell you to eat a protein, carbohydrate and fat at each meal or snack, but that combination might cause you indigestion. The real reason why a diet fails is that the diet was not a good fit for the person following it.

To create a good fit, you need to learn what your body wants and needs. You learn that by tuning in to your body and uncovering how it communicates with you. By paying attention, you will discover what, when, and how much to eat. In time, you will come to trust yourself and make choices based on what you know to be true for you. This is the essence of mindful eating.

Coming up, I will teach you how to tune into your body. I will show you how to eliminate all the noise from diet gurus, food manufacturers, and advertisers so you can hear the inner voice that wants to guide you. Once you are able to do that, your relationship with food changes and you will be on your way to permanent weight loss. With practice, you will learn to make the right choices for you at the right time, and some of those choices might surprise you. Let me give you an example from my own life.

I typically do not eat, or even enjoy, red meat, but I had an occasion when my body was "asking" for it. I had been attending a full-day conference. It was very busy and very exhausting. As the day came to an end, I noticed I was starting to feel under the weather. I thought I might be catching a cold. My colleagues wanted to go out to dinner, but I decided to return to my hotel room and order room service. Before looking at the menu I asked myself what my body wanted, and a picture of a hamburger popped into my head. The image surprised me, but I went with it.

I picked up the phone, called room service and asked for a burger. The person on the other end of the phone asked me which of the many burgers on the menu I wanted. I told her I simply wanted a burger. Nothing else. No fries. No chips. Just the burger. She was a bit confused (I guess people don't usually order that way) but placed my order anyway. When the burger arrived, it came with other items on the plate, but I ignored them. I bit into the burger, and it was surprisingly delicious. I ate it slowly and mindfully, curious as to why my body wanted this food at this time. After I finished, I felt a bit better. By the time morning came, I was completely restored. I can't explain it, but my body knew it needed whatever a burger would provide. I listened, and my body responded in kind. This is a great example of how listening to my body, rather than some prescribed rule about what I should or should not eat, served me well.

Listening to your body will serve you well too. Sometimes cravings, like the one I had for a hamburger, are messages from your body that something is missing. I encourage you to honor your cravings. However, if you find yourself eating hamburgers three times a day for several days in a row, there might be something else going on. You might want to talk with someone about your cravings. Maybe see a health care professional to find out if something is out of balance. Or a psychologist if your craving is emotional. If you just like burgers, watch the movie *Supersize Me*, which is about a guy who ate fast food for every meal for a month. It might just scare you straight.

The approach offered here does away with the dieting mentality so you can learn to trust yourself. By applying mindfulness, you will decide what foods and amounts are right for you. This approach will create a new flexible relationship to food and eating. You will learn to seek out the right type, quality, and quantity of food for you and no longer be handcuffed by diet rules and regulations. You will be able to dine out with friends, try new recipes, and even skip a meal or two if you are not hungry. You will learn how to manage your emotions without eating so that a bad day at the office or a fight with your significant other won't send you straight to the fridge. Eating mindfully and coping with your emotions without turning to food is, in the end, the best way to achieve healthy and permanent weight loss.

AND NOW FOR SOME BAD NEWS

I hope by now you are starting to get excited about the prospect of learning a new way to be with food that can end your weight struggle once and for all. I am excited for you. I know that as I learned and incorporated mindfulness into my eating, everything about my relationship to food and eating changed for the better. I am optimistic that the same can be true for you. But I must tell you the truth. This will take work!

Overeating and being overweight represent a set of unbalanced and unhealthy patterns that developed over a long period of time, perhaps even a lifetime. For you, overeating may have started in childhood. If you experienced some sort of trauma, such as the loss of a parent, divorce, or worse, you may have reached for food for comfort. As children, we have few skills to cope with pain, so eating might have been the only way to soothe the ache.

Family habits also form unhealthy eating patterns which lead to excess weight. If you had parents who were overweight, preferred the couch to a bike, called the local fast food joint their personal chef, or used food as a coping mechanism themselves, you may have learned your poor habits from them. Children model what they see. Who were your food role models?

Maybe your weight problem didn't start until later in life when you were faced with disappointments you didn't know how to deal with, or unwelcome changes in your body resulting in weight gain.

Regardless of why you are overweight or overeating, I am going to offer you a new set of patterns that will override your current ones. Success will happen, but it won't happen overnight. As you will discover, the more you practice these new behaviors and approaches, the faster you will see and feel results.

Think about this for a moment: you are where you are because of what you've done. We are the sum total of our choices. You may have had the best of intentions and I am sure you really tried your hardest. There is no guilt here. You haven't failed for lack of trying. You failed because what you chose to do just didn't work. Einstein is credited with saying that the definition of insanity is doing the same thing over again and expecting different results.

Now, I'm not saying any of us is insane, but what I am saying is that if we keep repeating what we've been doing, we will keep getting the same outcome. In other words, if you keep going on diets expecting to lose weight and keep it off, you will fail. If you keep reaching for a carton of ice cream thinking it will fix what ails you, you will be disappointed. If you want a different outcome, you must do something different. It's time for something new. It's time for mindful eating.

Through the five steps you will do in this version of my TAME Your Appetite programs, you will find and depend upon the wisdom you already have within you to create gradual changes in your eating and lifestyle patterns. You will no longer repeat the diet mistakes of the past. I suspect that deep down inside, you always knew that diets don't work, but you felt as if you had no other choice if you wanted to lose weight. The same thing is probably true about your emotional life. You know that chocolate doesn't mend a broken heart, but when you are grieving, it feels as if the creamy sweetness helps.

At its core, this program is about self-acceptance, self-care, and developing ways to meet your needs (all of them—physical and emotional) in healthy ways. Ultimately, you will develop a more natural, balanced relationship with food that leads you to make better choices in all you do.

A BIG WIN FOR YOU!

When you incorporate the 5 Steps into your daily life, you will experience much more than just weight loss. The tools and new behaviors I introduce will benefit other areas of your life too.

Because mindfulness meditation is the foundation of this program, you will get all the benefits that meditation has to offer, beyond taming your food issues. A regular mindfulness meditation practice has been associated with a reduction in stress and anxiety, an improvement in mood, lower blood pressure, less pain, improved relationships, and improved overall health. My clients have told me that they sleep better, have more energy, are more patient with their kids, and enjoy their spouses more after just a few weeks of applying mindfulness to their lives. Imagine how much better you will feel and how much more you will enjoy your life when you too experience these benefits.

Are you ready to begin? Or perhaps you feel like my client Gail did when she first heard about mindfulness. Luckily for her, she gave it a try.

Gail sank deep into the green leather of my office couch, placed her hands over her face and wept. Between sobs she told me how, once again, she regained the weight she dieted to lose. At forty-two years old, she felt as if she would never "conquer this problem" (her words) and felt resigned to "being fat" (again her words) for the rest of her life.

I could feel her pain as she described the week-long binge she fell into after getting some bad news. Bingeing in response to bad news was a pattern Gail had developed in childhood. The middle child of a single mother and absent alcoholic father, she grew up with plenty of bad news. Not having many resources, her mother used food as a way to soothe the pain. She would keep hard candies and small chocolates in her purse and whenever one of her kids was upset about something, she handed them a candy and reassured them that everything would be alright. Gail followed her mother's tradition and also kept candy in her purse, desk drawer, and glove compartment. She was never more than an arm's length from her stash.

What Gail hadn't learned yet was to be present in the company of bad news without reacting by eating sweets. Fortunately, she was about to learn mindfulness.

After she told me the story of her binge, I offered her an option.

I asked, "What if I could teach you how to respond differently when you got bad news? Not a different course of action or another way to feel, but rather, a way to be present with the discomfort without having to do anything about it?"

Gail raised her head from her hands and looked at me as if I had lost my mind. Before she could say anything, I added, "What if I could teach you a tool that would allow you to acknowledge and explore the bad news in such a way that you didn't feel the need to eat candy in response to it?"

Now I had her attention. She dabbed her eyes dry and gently nodded her head. And so began Gail's journey to mindfulness meditation and mindful eating.

Now it's your turn to join me in a new adventure with food and eating.

A WORD ABOUT WEIGHT LOSS AND WEIGHING YOURSELF

TAME Your Appetite is a non-diet approach to weight management. It is not a quick weight-loss program. Some people lose weight with this approach; others do not. Some initially gain weight when they discard previous restrictions and (mistakenly) replace it with permission to eat with abandon. If you are following this approach for weight loss, the more you practice the techniques and utilize the tools, the greater your chance for weight loss success.

If weight loss is your goal, I recommend that you weigh yourself no more than once a week while following the steps. More than that can be counterproductive. Less than that is even better. If you do weigh yourself, I suggest you do so with an attitude of curiosity and acceptance. Use your scale as a feedback tool and nothing more. Please do not use the number on the scale as a way to condemn yourself or this approach if you do not see a number you like. Focus your energy on the behaviors, attitudes and habits that you are changing rather than the number on the scale. If you do that, I believe you will be pleasantly surprised. Stephanie was.

Stephanie was a daily weigher. Every morning she would get on the scale. If she travelled, she took her scale with her. Sometimes she weighed herself twice a day. I asked her why she weighed herself so often and she told me that she was afraid that if she didn't know her weight, she would keep eating. On days when she felt she ate too much, she weighed herself in the evening to see how much damage she had done.

When I asked Stephanie how this routine worked for her, she sadly replied with, "Look at me," as she pointed to her 200-pound body. That began a conversation about how she felt about herself and her body and the role the frequent weighing might be playing.

She told me seeing the number on the scale did not have the positive influence she hoped it would. She told me that she expected that when the number was higher than she wanted it to be it would encourage her to eat less, but that rarely happened. More often, her disappointment in seeing the larger number led her to eat more because she was angry and upset. This would be followed by an even more stringent diet than the one she was already on. When the number was lower, she confessed she also ate more.

When I asked why, she answered, "The lower number means I've been good and now I can splurge a little."

It didn't take long for Stephanie to see the error in her ways. I asked her if she would be willing to not weigh herself while she was working with me. Trusting that I knew what I was doing, she agreed, but admitted that having the scale in her home would be hard to resist.

We came up with a plan that her husband would take the scale to his office for the duration of the mindful eating program. Stephanie was terrified at the idea of not weighing herself but, with my encouragement and the love of her husband, she agreed to give it a try. Over the next few months, Stephanie focused her attention on the approach and new skills I was teaching her. We measured her successes by how many times she meditated and how often she tuned in to her body for guidance, rather than by how much she may have weighed. As we approached the end of the formal program, Stephanie told her husband to keep the scale. She was happy with the changes she was noticing in her mood, energy level and waistband, and no longer needed to know the numbers.

Stephanie's improvements are an excellent example of what could happen for you as you learn how to TAME Your Appetite. If disappointment in seeing a higher number on a scale leads you to eat more, that can change. If you eat when you are angry, you can learn other ways to handle that emotion. If you tend to put yourself on stringent diets to gain control over your eating, I can show you a better way. By embracing the tenets and practices of mindful eating that follow, you, too, can experience a sense of self-love that is not dependent on any number on any scale.

MINDFUL BITE:
Every bite is an opportunity to practice mindful eating.

Chapter Two
Becoming Mindful

Washing the dishes to wash the dishes.

Thich Nhat Hanh

As we begin your journey to mindful eating, I'd like to take a moment to share with you how I discovered mindfulness and mindful eating, how it helped me improve my relationship with food, and how I use what I learned to help my clients.

MY STRUGGLE

They say you teach what you need to learn. I have found this to be true. After twenty years as a practicing psychologist, I am still learning by teaching. Not in the traditional sense of standing in front of a classroom (although, I do that too for college and psychology grad students). No, rather I "teach" by guiding my clients through the trials and tribulations of their lives. And I learn what to teach by being a student first. I was (and still am) always reading, taking classes, listening to lectures, and going to conferences. I am motivated to continue learning for two reasons. First, to become a better clinician and second, to become a better version of me. And it is here where my story begins.

From the winter of 2015 through the summer of 2018, I was in a free fall. My family was besieged by death, illness, and constant change. I spent most of my days helping my sister take care of our aging parents who lived 3,000 miles away from me. I travelled to them almost every other month, taking the red eye from Los Angeles after a full day of clients and flying back on another red eye just in time to return to my practice. To say it was stressful is an understatement. To say that I abandoned my own self-care in favor of my family's needs would be the truth. As a consequence, I suffered.

Oh, and did I mention I was going through menopause at the same time? Seriously! Here I was, counseling my clients to take care of themselves and forgetting to do the same for myself. I was out of shape, gaining weight, and losing sleep. The good news is that because I am always a student first, I would stop at the bookstores in every airport I frequented and buy something new. By doing that, I learned about mindfulness, mindful eating, and the work of Dr. Jean Kristeller. I was intrigued. The research was showing how mindfulness, especially mindfulness meditation, could help with stress. Woo-hoo! Sign me up.

As I dove deeper into mindfulness and mindful eating (my career had focused on eating disorders and emotional overeating, so I was naturally inclined towards this material), I learned about Dr. Kristeller's professional training program for eating disorder specialists to teach mindfulness-based eating awareness. I applied, was accepted, and began my professional training in MB-EAT. Here's where my teaching became what I needed to learn.

One of the requirements to become an MB-EAT Instructor was to develop a daily meditation practice. So, I got books, audio recordings, and took classes to learn the skill. I participated in my training program to become an MB-EAT instructor and, along the way, recognized that the mindfulness habits I was being taught to teach are habits that I myself needed. So, I decided to take a year to apply what I was learning to myself to see what changes would occur. WOW! If I knew then what I know now, I would have done this mindfulness thing decades ago!

Once I started incorporating mindfulness meditation and mindful eating skills into my daily life, things improved in ways I hadn't anticipated. The first thing I noticed was that I was lessening my stress eating. This change happened even though the level of stress in my life had not. I was still dealing with the same issues as I had previously, but now I was not reaching for food as a coping mechanism.

I was also sleeping better. Insomnia had become a constant companion. I could fall asleep easily, but I could not stay asleep. Suddenly I was sleeping through the night and when I awoke, I had more energy and focus. The more I practiced mindfulness meditation and mindful eating, the better things got. What was happening for me was consistent with the research from Dr. Kristeller. Her studies showed that the people who practiced the meditations and tools the most had the best success. Slowly I started to mention mindfulness, mindfulness meditation, and mindful eating to my clients. I directed them towards resources I thought would help them. I noticed that those who used the resources started to report the same benefits I was experiencing myself. I knew I was on the right track.

Jessica was one of the first clients to whom I mentioned mindfulness meditation. She had a propensity for sweets but was not overweight. She also had a lot of anxiety. Massive amounts. So much that her work as a court reporter was starting to suffer. I brought up the subject by simply asking her if she ever meditated. She said she had on and off for years but could never quite get the hang of it. She thought she was doing it "wrong" because she couldn't turn her mind off. I explained to Jessica that turning one's mind off is not the goal of mindfulness meditation, nor could it be. Our minds work 24/7. We can't stop that, but what we can do is learn to observe where our thoughts go. By learning how to observe our thoughts, we can exercise more control over our responses to them. And by learning to exercise more control over our responses, our lives become better. Jessica was intrigued and a bit apprehensive for her first lesson in mindfulness meditation.

YOUR INTRODUCTION TO MINDFULNESS

Now let me introduce you to mindfulness and mindfulness meditation. The practice of mindfulness is a powerful one because it gets us out of automatic habits and reactions and helps create different responses to what is happening around us. With mindfulness, we have the opportunity to create new, healthier habits that serve us better. Mindfulness brings automatic reactions more under conscious control, thus allowing our innate wisdom to take charge rather than having our old habitual patterns at the helm. This makes us more aware, in positive ways, of our experiences. How does that happen? Let's start by incorporating mindfulness into your life right now to find out.

Find a window you can look out of for several minutes without being disturbed. Take a seat near the window and settle into it. Place your feet on the floor, your hands in your lap and take three slow deep breaths. This is centering yourself. Once you are centered, look out the window. Just look. What do you see? Buildings? Cars? Trees? Birds? People? What colors do you see? Are any of the colors particularly bright? Anything unusual happening? Just observe. If your mind wanders while you are looking out the window, that's fine. No worries. As soon as you notice this happening, acknowledge it and go back to looking out the window. Is it day or night? Are there streetlamps? Traffic? When a few minutes are up, bring your attention back into the room and check in with yourself.

How was that experience? Did you enjoy it? Were you bored? Do you feel more alert and present? Is anything different? One more big question: in what way is how you just looked out the window different than how you usually look out? Some people describe noticing more than usual when they do this exercise. Others say that they have looked out the same window for years and never before noticed certain details. A bird's nest, for example. A new street sign. Vibrant colors. More activity than they expected. They noticed more during this exercise because typically, when people look out a window, it's a quick glance and onto the next thing. All of this "noticing," and all of these "observations," are demonstrations of mindfulness. Beginning today, you can bring mindfulness into your life by simply choosing to pay more attention. And you can do this with everyday ordinary experiences.

The quote at the start of this chapter is attributed to Thich Nhat Hanh, a Vietnamese Buddhist monk who lectured around the world on Buddhist principles and philosophies. He told a story of when he was a novice monk and tasked with washing dishes. They had no soap—only ashes, husks, and pots of hot water. He explained that at the monastery, he learned the value of washing dishes just for the sake of washing them. He came to understand that while washing the dishes, that is all one should be doing. Meaning that, when you are washing dishes, put your full attention on that very act. Don't think about anything else. Don't hurry through the activity to get to the next one. Just wash the dishes. In doing so, he discovered a peacefulness and sense of presence that was astonishing to him. By focusing all of his attention on washing the dishes, he was able to reflect on the value and joy of living one moment of life at a time.

Think about Thich Nhat Hanh the next time you are faced with a sink full of dishes. Or a load of laundry. Or while walking the dog, brushing your teeth, or taking a shower. Approach each of these activities as if it were the only thing in the world that requires your attention in the moment. See if you discover the joy that comes from such focus.

Sometimes, I like to practice mindfulness when I am at a traffic light. Instead of feeling impatient, I take a breath and look around. I see cars, storefronts, and people. I hear traffic, horns, radios, conversations. I give myself the gift of that moment. And then when the light changes and traffic moves again, I am calmer, more centered, less rushed. I find myself doing this in line at the grocery store and when I am waiting in the dentist chair. This is mindfulness in everyday life. I call these "mindful moments," and when I fill my day with many of these moments, my day goes much smoother. I believe yours will too. Give it a try!

Connor, a quick-witted, charismatic, forty-five-year-old trial attorney, challenged me on the idea of practicing mindfulness every day. He thought the idea was too "woo-woo" for him. He equated it with being a navel-gazing hippie. Having been a lawyer myself, I thought of one place where practicing mindfulness would be especially helpful—in court. In my day, we used to rush to court, petrified to be late and receive the judge's wrath. Instead, we got there on time and then sat around for hours until our cases were called. We used to refer to that phenomena as the "hurry up and wait."

I asked Connor if the old adage "hurry up and wait" still applied. He tilted his head back and with a hearty belly laugh said, "Oh boy does it!"

"Great," I responded. "Let's use it."

I asked Connor to practice mindfulness the next time he was in court. I asked him to spend the time he was waiting around to observe his surroundings. No texting. No typing on his laptop. Just observing. At first, he resisted, saying he used his courtroom down time to work. I acknowledged that (I used to do that too) and requested if, for one day, he could humor me and try mindfulness. His fellow program participants urged him on, so he agreed.

I eagerly awaited the next program session to hear what happened, as did the other participants. As soon as he came in the door, they bombarded him with questions about court. Always happy to take the spotlight, Connor regaled the group with the events of that day. He began by describing the courtroom in great detail. He admitted that he had been there hundreds of times, but never noticed the statues or pictures that were scattered about. He got the group laughing when he told of the wardrobes some of the other lawyers were wearing. References to the movie *My*

Cousin Vinny abounded. He mimicked the judge's East Coast accent and the bailiff's walk. Then he got serious.

He said that because he was paying full attention in court, he felt better prepared when his turn came to argue his motion. He heard the opposing counsel's position more clearly and could refute it with greater ease. By being more present, he felt more confident. When the judge ruled in his favor, he thought to himself, *Maybe Doc* (he calls me Doc) *is right about this mindfulness.* The group applauded when he finished. Hands clapped in high fives and Connor took his seat, eager to learn how else mindfulness might help him.

BENEFITS OF MINDFULNESS FOR YOUR HEALTH AND OVERALL WELL-BEING

As previously mentioned, there are many reasons to incorporate mindfulness into your life besides changing your weight. Mindfulness has been known to decrease stress, lower blood pressure, reduce depression and its accompanying rumination, lessen anxiety, diminish body aches and pains, limit distractions, ease emotional reactions, increase self-observation, improve relationship skills, heighten relationship satisfaction, enhance self-expression, increase positive moods, boost memory, enrich focus, and increase immune functioning. We will explore these benefits in Step Five.

As you will see, a daily meditation practice and a mindful approach to everyday living can have miraculous-like effects in your life. To begin, let's take a closer look at the principles of mindfulness and mindfulness meditation in general.

THE PRINCIPLES OF MINDFULNESS

There are seven principles of mindfulness. They are non-judging, patience, non-striving, letting go, acceptance, beginner's mind, and trust. Each one plays a role in mindful eating and mindfulness meditation. How they do so will become apparent as you move through the program. Let's start with a brief look at how these principles will be applied.

- Trust, patience, and non-striving will be used to support your transition from your old eating habits to your new mindful ones. You will be encouraged to relax into this process rather than forcing it to happen so that you won't have to try hard to gain results.
- Beginner's mind will be used to avoid the trap of thinking that a slip into mindless eating, a full-blown binge, or a lapse in your meditation practice will negate all your efforts and be a signal to give up yet again.
- Letting go, non-judging, and acceptance will help reduce weight-related fear and anxiety by cultivating a point-of-view that minimizes reactivity and prevents the urge to trash this approach and sign up for another diet.

There are three other aspects of mindfulness that will also play an important role in the changes you will be making. The first is self-compassion, which is a form of loving self-kindness. If you tend to be impatient, punitive, and self-critical, demanding more of yourself than you do of others, self-compassion will be an important ally in this journey. When you approach yourself with kindness rather than criticism, you will find that you can do and be more.

Impermanence is another aspect of mindfulness which teaches us that everything (including our weight) is temporary. Excess weight can be seen as a transient state that can pass. The same is true for a binge or emotional eating episode. They don't last forever. Accepting impermanence will help end the, *I've blown it, this will never work, so I might as well eat it all* mentality.

Lastly, the idea of non-attachment to outcomes can reduce the suffering that impatience causes and will allow you to let this process unfold in the way that is best for you and your body. For example, when you are on a diet, I suspect you decide your success based on what the scale says. If you lost weight that week, you were "good;" if you didn't, you were "bad." Being attached to the number on the scale may cause you to lose sight of the many other successes that actually occurred that week. For example, maybe you didn't eat when you weren't hungry, or you stopped when you were full. Maybe you said no to seconds, meditated daily, or expressed your emotions instead of eating over them. Or perhaps you showed up for yourself in ways you might not have before. So even if the scale didn't reflect a weight loss, a review of those other successes could motivate you to keep going. All you have to do is let go of your attachment to the number on the scale and look instead to the bigger picture.

WHAT IS MINDFULNESS MEDITATION?

Now let's turn our attention to mindfulness meditation. While rooted in Buddhist traditions, mindfulness meditation is not a religious practice and you do not need to be Buddhist to benefit from it. Nor is mindfulness meditation about clearing the mind or going into a trance. It is also not merely another form of relaxation. Mindfulness meditation is a practice which allows us to gain moment-to-moment insights into the activities of our minds and bodies. We can use these insights to help ourselves see a situation more clearly and become open to new ways of responding. Being mindful simply means seeing the current moment without judgment. It is an intentional act of present-moment awareness without attachment to any particular outcome. By paying attention to the here and now and watching each moment pass, we can begin to see a situation or problem more fully and become awakened to a new solution which allows us to choose a different response or action.

Let me explain how this applies to eating and weight loss. According to Buddhist tradition, life is suffering. We suffer because we are attached to outcomes. We suffer when we diet because we crave weight loss—the outcome of dieting. The more we strive for this outcome, the more we suffer. Mindfulness meditation is designed to enhance our ability to respond to the psychological and physical states associated with eating with self-compassion and acceptance rather than with mindless attachment to the numbers on a scale.

Since mindfulness meditation is the central ingredient in this mindfulness-based approach, it is important to develop and maintain a consistent meditation practice. By practicing mindfulness meditation, you will draw your attention to the present moment and allow yourself to be patient with whatever is happening. You will learn to let go of a desired outcome (such as losing a certain number of pounds each week) and instead accept whatever outcome there is. When you do that, you change your relationship to your experience of eating which, in time, will change your eating habits.

If you are still unsure about meditation, and its origins in Buddhism, maybe you can relate to Hillary.

"But I'm not Buddhist," Hillary declared when I introduced the origins of mindfulness meditation at a recent introductory workshop. "I can't do this! I am a nice Jewish girl from Brooklyn. How can you even suggest this?"

I, too, am a nice Jewish girl from Brooklyn, so I explained to Hillary that all major religions, including Judaism, practice some form of meditation. Still, one does not need to be religious or even spiritual to gain the benefits a meditation practice can offer. Seeing that Hillary is still not sure about "all this Buddhist stuff," I assured her that religion has nothing to do with the meditation work we do in mindful eating. I asked her to keep an open mind for the duration of the workshop and to join me as I led the group in short introductory practice.

I took Hillary and the other workshop attendees through a brief general meditation that asked them to simply focus their attention on their breath. At the conclusion of the meditation, I asked for feedback.

Hillary's hand shot up and she asked, "Where was Buddha? Did I miss him?"

I responded, "Hillary, there was no mention of Buddha. The only role Buddha plays is a historical one."

"So, that's it?" she continued. "All I have to do is pay attention to my breath and I'm meditating?"

"That's it," I said.

"Well, then why didn't you say that in the first place?" The attendees and I couldn't help but laugh as she said that.

MINDFUL BITE:

Mindfulness is simply being present with purpose and intention.

Chapter Three
TAME Your Appetite – The 5-Step Plan

When eating an elephant, take one bite at a time.
CREIGHTON W. ADAMS, JR.

Welcome to the 5-Step program to get you on your way to a new relationship with food and a healthy body weight. These steps are based on my complete, *TAME Your Appetite: The Art of Mindful Eating* workshops and coaching programs and give you the opportunity to experience what such a powerful program can do for you.

MINDFUL EATING IS THE SOLUTION

Mindful eating offers a solution to your weight and food battles by increasing the pleasure and satisfaction you get from eating. With mindful eating, you will discover that you naturally eat smaller amounts of food and, over time, make wiser choices about what, when, and how much to eat. You will be drawn to options that lead to good health and weight loss and that change long-standing eating habits and patterns.

WHAT IS MINDFUL EATING?

- Mindful eating quite simply means eating with awareness and intention so you can really taste the food you are eating, enjoy it more, and be satisfied with less. When you eat mindfully, you:
- Focus your attention on the food you are about to eat;
- Check in with how hungry or full you are;
- Observe the food in front of you, noticing its appearance, scent, and texture;
- Appreciate how the food got to you, acknowledging the farmers, manufacturers, transportation vehicles, stock clerks, cashiers, cooks, and others who participated in getting it to you;
- Eat your food slowly, paying attention to how it tastes and feels in your mouth, noticing when and if the taste changes;

- Check-in periodically with your hunger and fullness signals; and
- Stop when you notice that you have had enough and feel satisfied.

This may seem complicated, excessive, and even tedious, but I promise, as you establish mindful eating as your new eating pattern, all of this will become second nature. It will become how you eat, and your body will respond accordingly.

To illustrate mindful eating, I will now guide you through a very famous mindful eating exercise. This exercise is offered in mindfulness-based classes worldwide—even those not dealing with mindful eating. The reason it is so popular is because, in just a few minutes, you will begin to understand mindfulness in a way you never have before.

THE RAISIN EXERCISE

To do the Raisin Exercise, you will need four raisins. Place the raisins on a small plate or napkin and bring them to wherever you will be sitting to do this exercise. The Raisin Exercise is in the form of a meditation. Use the script below. Have someone read it to you or record it for yourself to make it easier to use. When you are ready, get comfortable in your chair and we'll begin.

THE RAISIN EXERCISE SCRIPT

Close your eyes and take two or three relaxed breaths. If you don't want to close your eyes, just shut them partially and let your gaze rest on the floor in front of you.

Become aware of your breath flowing in and flowing out. Notice your chest and stomach gently rising and falling with each breath. Take two or three more slow deep breaths.

Now, open your eyes and take one of the raisins. Look at it with curiosity, as if you have never seen a raisin before. Examine its folds and color.

Now close your eyes and, with your eyes shut, bring the raisin up to your nose and smell it.

Now touch the outside of your lips with the raisin.

Notice any thoughts or feelings that come up about raisins.

With your eyes still closed, place the raisin in your mouth, but do not chew it yet. Notice how it feels on your tongue. Move it around your mouth and notice any sensations.

Now begin to chew the raisin, noticing how the flavor changes as you bite into it.

Chew it very slowly, experiencing its taste and feel. Resist the urge to swallow it.

Notice any thoughts or feelings you have about eating this raisin.

Now, if you are ready, swallow it.

Are there any tastes lingering in your mouth? Be aware of any sensations in your body and in your mouth.

Recognize that your body has taken in the weight and food energy of this one raisin.

Now open your eyes and pick up another raisin.

Again, examine it and then close your eyes and smell it. Has anything changed? Is anything different?

Be aware of whatever thoughts and feelings are arising.

Place the raisin in your mouth, and again, experience this raisin first without chewing it and then by chewing it slowly, observing the taste and the texture.

Are there any similarities or differences with the first raisin?

Be aware, as much as you can, of any experiences of pleasure and satisfaction from this small morsel of food.

When you are ready to swallow, do so noticing the raisin going down the back of your throat.

Now open your eyes and pick up the third raisin. This time lead yourself through examining, smelling, eating, and savoring this raisin mindfully.

As you finish with the third raisin, what are you aware of?

Once again, open your eyes and look at the fourth raisin. You may choose to eat this raisin or not. Take a moment and be aware of how you are making this choice.

If you choose to eat the fourth raisin, again lead yourself through the practice. If not, then with your eyes closed, simply be aware of your breath, thoughts, feelings, and sensations in your mouth and elsewhere.

Now bring your awareness gently back to your breath. Take two or three more relaxing breaths and when you are ready, open your eyes.

Congratulations. You are a mindful eater! Let's take a moment to reflect on your experience.

In doing this exercise, it is quite common to have a wide range of reactions. Remember this was an introduction to eating mindfully and to treating food like a gourmet would, purely for the experience of eating. It is very likely that you have never eaten this way before and that you have never tasted a raisin as fully as you have in this exercise. What happened to you?

- Did you experience a sense of awe at the intense flavor of one raisin, whether it tasted good or bad to you?
- Were you surprised at the differences among raisins when eaten mindfully one by one?
- Were you satisfied from eating so few raisins?
- Did how you feel about raisins change?
- What thoughts came to mind as you ate the raisins?
- What emotions did you have?
- Were there any surprises?
- How might this experience of eating a raisin help with your eating or weight issues?

Remember this experience as you move forward in your journey. You do not need to eat everything the way you ate the raisins, but from time to time, doing so can be quite enjoyable.

In one of my early TAME Your Appetite programs, one participant, Evelyn, refused to do the raisin exercise. As I distributed the raisins, she proclaimed, "I hate raisins!" The group got quiet and waited nervously to see what I would do.

I turned toward Evelyn and very kindly said, "No worries, you can observe as the group does this meditation and then you can do it at home with whatever food you prefer."

Relieved that she did not have to eat any raisins, Evelyn sat back in her chair and watched. While I was moving around the room, I told Evelyn that she could participate in the exercise even if she didn't eat the raisin, if she wanted to. Evelyn refused.

"That's fine," I replied as I handed the woman sitting next to her some raisins.

"Okay," Evelyn said. "I can hold them."

"Wonderful," I responded and placed four raisins onto the napkin in front of her.

When everyone had their raisins, we began.

The group settled into their breathing and picked up the first raisin. I instructed the group to experience the raisin with all their senses. Evelyn did everything I suggested except put the raisin in her mouth. When the group moved onto the second raisin, so did Evelyn. Again, she smelled it, felt it, and placed it near her lips, but did not eat it. The group went on to lead themselves through the exercise with the third raisin on their own. This time I noticed that Evelyn placed the raisin in her mouth. I could see her suck on it, bite it gently, chew it completely, and then swallow. When given the choice to eat the fourth raisin, Evelyn picked another one up and led herself once more through the meditation.

At the end, when the group discussed their experiences, Evelyn surprised all of us when she said that it turns out she doesn't hate raisins. When asked for details, Evelyn revealed that she thought she didn't like raisins because her mother used to put raisins into a particular noodle dish served at holidays. Evelyn concluded that she didn't like the noodle dish, but raisins were delicious!

If you don't like raisins, you don't have to use them for this exercise. Choose something else such as grapes, blueberries, or olives. The point of this meditation is to have the experience of really tasting a particular food. To be present with it via all your senses so you can see, feel, and taste what you might miss if you ate the food mindlessly.

With the Raisin Exercise behind us, let me introduce you to the 5 Steps.

THE 5 STEPS

This specific version of my *TAME Your Appetite* program is made up of five steps. I will explain briefly what each step entails and in the next five chapters we will explore them one by one in greater depth.

Step One is establishing a daily meditation practice. Meditation is the foundation of this program, as well as my complete *TAME Your Appetite* curriculum. Research into mindful eating has proven that the more you engage in a daily meditation practice, the more successful you will be in reducing unnecessary eating, especially binge and emotional eating. If you are new to meditation or feel nervous about the whole idea, don't worry. I will help you every step of the way.

The second step is cultivating your Inner Wisdom. By Inner Wisdom, I mean your body's own innate understanding of what it needs, when it needs it, and how much it needs. By cultivating your Inner Wisdom, you will learn to eat when you are hungry, stop when you are full, eat the right foods in the right amounts for you, and truly enjoy yourself. Your relationship to food, to eating, and to your self will change as you get more in touch with your Inner Wisdom. It is these changes that will lead you to a healthy weight and peace with food.

Step Three teaches you how to balance your eating habits with reliable, scientifically established nutritional information which I call Outer Guidance. Outer Guidance is information which you will consider as you decide what foods to eat. Outer Guidance is not a diet or set of rules that you must follow. Instead, it is a state of mind where you become curious about the nutritional value of food and how foods affect your body. It is about learning to appreciate the health benefits some foods provide and grasping the detrimental effects other foods may have. The truth is, calories count, some foods are more beneficial for your health than others, and certain foods may be downright harmful. By cultivating your Outer Guidance, you will learn to make informed choices.

The fourth step addresses emotional eating. Emotional eating is eating in response to feelings. It's using food as a coping mechanism when you feel sad, angry, lonely, or any other host of emotions. Eating in response to your emotions can lead to the consumption of excess calories which in turn leads to excess weight. For many people, just ending emotional eating can lead them to the weight loss they seek. This step will provide tools for you to explore your emotions without turning to food.

Step Five expands mindfulness to the rest of your life. Think of it as a bonus step that will guide you to healing much more than your relationship to food. We will explore the benefits of mindfulness meditation for stress, anxiety, depression, physical pain and insomnia. You will learn how to use mindfulness in everyday life, and I'll give you tips on how to get good at it.

Before we jump into the 5 Steps in more detail, let's look at some of the obstacles that might get in the way as you get ready to embrace mindful eating.

OBSTACLES

Starting something new can be intimidating. Faced with changing how we do things can be frightening. In response to such intimidation and fear, we often find ourselves resisting the very things that would serve us best. We express that resistance by finding reasons for why what we are about to embark on cannot work. We are in fact creating obstacles to our own success. Below are six common "reasons" (aka obstacles) I hear all the time when I introduce the ideas associated with mindful eating. Let's look at each of them and see how you can move them out of your way.

OBSTACLE #1: FEAR OF ROCKING THE BOAT

I will start with this obstacle because this is the one I hear most often, especially from people who are in relationships or living with others. Taking a mindful approach to food and eating will most likely be different from how you and your loved ones typically eat. For example, you will be spending more attention on your food, perhaps eating more slowly than before, which can sometimes raise eyebrows. Being different takes courage. The way to manage this obstacle is to let people know ahead of time what you are doing. Tell them that you are taking a new approach to health and weight management and that you will be paying more attention to how, what and when you eat. Invite them to join you. Once you get the hang of mindful eating, you will be able to eat in any situation and not draw attention to yourself. Mindful eating is actually a private venture and unless you point it out to others, it can be done in relative anonymity.

OBSTACLE #2: I LOVE FOOD

This obstacle, you will find, is no obstacle at all. In fact, with mindful eating you will enjoy eating even more. You will come to appreciate quality over quantity and find that your meals and snacks are more pleasurable than before. That's one of the gifts of mindful eating. What this obstacle may be really speaking to is the idea that you want to eat what you want to eat without having to pay attention. Remember, we call that mindless eating.

Here's the truth: you can continue mindless eating if you want to, just do it mindfully! In other words, with full attention and purpose. For example, you have had a bad day and you want to eat an entire bag of chips. Okay. Have the chips. Just acknowledge that this is what you are doing. Make it a conscious choice and enjoy. Pour the chips into a beautiful bowl. Sit down on your favorite chair and savor each crispy, greasy morsel. Mindful eating is about loving food and the joy of eating. You don't have to give those up.

OBSTACLE #3: I HAVE TOO MANY THINGS TO DO; I DON'T HAVE TIME FOR THIS

Being busy is an American pastime. Between work, school, family, home, and hobbies, it can feel like there are never enough hours in the day. So, for some, maybe you, practicing mindful eating and its companion, mindfulness meditation, become more of what we "must" do. To some extent, this is true. And yet, if we are honest with ourselves, we can admit that we do find the time to do the things we want to do. The answer to this obstacle is to make practicing mindful eating and establishing a meditation practice something you want to do. In the beginning, it takes time and effort for sure, but it's worth it.

After a while, mindful eating and meditating become second nature and require little exertion at all. Also, people report that when they add meditation to their schedule, they find they are more efficient, more relaxed, and better able to get other tasks done than before. That sounds like a win-win to me.

OBSTACLE #4: MEDITATION IS TOO HARD; I CAN'T QUIET MY MIND

People tell me that they can't meditate. They say it is too hard. They feel that because they can't quiet their minds, they are doing something wrong. They quit before they get the benefits meditation has to offer. I am here to tell you that meditation can seem hard. Our minds wander. We become bored. We may even fear what our thoughts might reveal. These statements are all true and yet they do not need to be reasons to shy away from meditating. As you will learn, the goal of meditation is not to silence the mind, but rather, to observe it . . . to be with it. To develop a curiosity about how your mind works. To observe what thoughts it thinks, even if those thoughts are disturbing.

Over time you will discover that troubling thoughts become just thoughts and your mind does settle down. Not completely, but enough so that you feel as if you have some control. You'll have some peace of mind. I urge you not to give up if you feel as if meditation is too hard. Go through the motions. Set time aside and sit. Just sit. Nothing else. If all you do during that time is mentally prepare your shopping list, that's fine. Just keep sitting. Eventually you will find yourself tuning into your mind a bit more. Your focus will turn more towards your breath and then, without you even realizing it, you are a meditator.

OBSTACLE #5: I CAN'T SIT FOR THAT LONG

Not being able to sit for long is something I can relate to. Posture is an important part of meditating and finding the right position for you may take some time. (I'm still working on it.) Many meditation teachers recommend you sit slightly forward and upright in a chair with your feet on the ground and your hands in your lap. Others suggest sitting on a cushion with your knees slightly below your hips and your feet crossed at the ankles. Others prefer meditation benches which allow for a kneeling position. Sitting still for several minutes (not to mention an hour as some meditators do) can be difficult, especially if you are not used to it. Your back may hurt. Your body may ache. You may itch. Your legs may tingle. You may feel fidgety. No worries. It's all okay. Just try different positions until you find what works best for you. If you need to move around while meditating, do so. You don't have to sit crossed legged in the lotus position to meditate. Even though we will talk about a "sitting" meditation practice, it is okay to practice lying down. For some people, that is the most comfortable. If you do lie down, try not to fall asleep. If you are on your bed and find yourself drifting off, move to the floor. Lie on a yoga mat or blanket. Practice with different positions until you find your favorite.

OBSTACLE #6: I CAN'T KEEP AT IT

The last obstacle we will address is the concern that you can't stay with this. As with any new habit or activity, it will take time to "get good" at mindful eating. Like the old joke about how to get to Carnegie Hall … you need to practice, practice, practice. While practice may make perfect, you do not need perfect practice. In other words, you don't have to mindfully eat all the time. You don't have to practice your meditation every day. It is what you do most of the time that makes the difference. Let go of the idea that you have to do this "perfectly" and just do it. If you get sidetracked, no worries, just start again. Your meditation practice of coming back to the breath when your mind wanders will teach you to do that. In fact, that is one of the reasons that meditation is the foundation of this program. Learning to start again is valuable. Learning to get back to your purpose (breathing, eating mindfully, etc.) as soon as you realize you have gone astray is what will make you successful in the long run. Go for it. Practice as much as you can. If you stop, start again and again and again. That's what Susanne did. She kept starting again until it clicked.

Susanne was one of my first mindful eating clients. She had been a dieter and emotional eater since her teens. She was convinced that nothing would change. When I introduced her to the idea of mindful eating, she said, "sure, why not?" Why not indeed?

We began by adding meditation to her daily routine. We changed nothing about her food or eating habits. For the first week, Susanne meditated every day for ten minutes. Then she didn't. Work got in the way. Then she was gone on business travel.

Weeks passed before I saw her again. When she returned, we began again, and again she practiced daily until she didn't. This on/off routine went on for months. Some weeks she'd practice twice, others four times, often just once. To help her see the value of meditation to her eating, I asked Susanne to pay attention to whether her eating and food choices were different on the days she meditated compared to the days she didn't. At first, she said there was no difference and then something changed. She realized that when she did her daily meditation practice, she ate less food at night (her usual binge time). When we explored why that was, she recognized that on those days, she felt less stressed. Less stress translated to less emotional eating for her. With this insight, Susanne found herself more able to start again each time her practice stalled. Eventually, she was able to practice six to seven times a week, knowing that if she got distracted by work or life, she could always start again.

I hope by now you are convinced and ready to start eating mindfully.

WHAT TO EXPECT FROM MINDFUL EATING

If you are brand new to mindful eating, you may be wondering what awaits you. Let's take a quick look at some of what is to come.

— THE GOOD NEWS —

PEACE WITH FOOD

The first benefit many people experience when they engage in mindful eating is noticing a sense of peace with food. The battle is over. With mindfulness, you give yourself permission to choose foods based on your preferences rather than some diet rule or dictate. With practice, you learn that you can trust yourself to make mindful choices based on your body's needs. That's peace.

Tia was especially interested in this benefit of mindful eating. "A compulsive dieter," as she describes herself, Tia was constantly at odds with herself, her body, and her appetite. She bounced between diets and binges her entire adult life. Approaching seventy, she was sure "this problem would never be solved."

I asked Tia a question similar to one I had learned from Dr. Kristeller: "What if a year from now you have lost weight. Maybe not as much as you wanted to lose, but you knew that what you lost was gone for good. How would you feel?"

Tia struggled with coming up with an answer because she didn't want to give up the dream of being "skinny."

I continued, "And, what if not only those pounds were gone for good, but you felt safe around food, you stopped chasing diets, you quit bingeing and finally felt comfortable in your body?"

She sat quietly thinking. "You mean, I might not be skinny, but the war would be over?"

I nodded, "Yes, the war would be over."

Tears formed in her eyes, and she said, "If I could live the rest of my life at peace with food, I would be happy."

Mindful eating is not a panacea for all that ails you. It is not a magic formula that will melt fat away, but it is a way of life that can restore health and well-being. It is an approach to food that can calm the nerves, reconnect you to your body, and establish a set of habits that can last a lifetime.

WEIGHT LOSS

In addition, as you become more tuned into mindful eating and establish your meditation practice, your body will naturally release whatever excess weight you might be holding on to. This happens because as a mindful eater you actually become a pickier eater, choosing quality over quantity. As a consequence, you will naturally eat less while feeling more satisfied. This change results in weight loss as the body returns to where it needs to be to be healthy. This weight loss may happen quickly, slowly, or somewhere in between.

One caveat—for some people initially there may be no weight loss or maybe even some weight gain. I see this happen when people remove their previously held food restrictions and indulge in all their formerly forbidden foods. For them, the idea of not dieting translates to permission to binge. This is an understandable reaction to years (even decades) of dietary deprivation. If this happens to you, don't worry. Eventually, you'll get over this behavior and balanced mindful eating will prevail.

Now let's look at the "maybe not-so-good news."

—THE MAYBE NOT-SO-GOOD NEWS—

To be fair, there are some changes that may come along with mindful eating that may be upsetting to you. These changes are actually good news, but at first you might not think so. Let's take a look at them so you don't get derailed and abandon your mindful eating practice.

NO MORE MINDLESS EATING

To eat mindfully means that you will no longer be able to eat mindlessly because you now know too much. Mindless eating is a habit which many of us engage in as a way to escape life's pressures and avoid difficult situations and emotions. Zoning out in front of the TV with a carton of ice cream is the way some people spend their evenings. When you eat mindlessly, you swallow spoons full of ice cream with barely a taste. You have little memory of having eaten the ice cream at all. The only real evidence are the drip stains on the front of your t-shirt!

To eat mindfully means that you no longer zone out with a carton of ice cream. At first, you may think this is unacceptable. You may believe that giving up mindless eating is a big deal and one you're not sure you want to commit to. I understand. When people hear me talk about giving up mindless eating, they think that means I am saying they must give up the foods they eat mindlessly or that they must stop doing other things when they eat. Not true. I am not saying you can never eat ice cream from the carton again or that you can never again eat in front of the TV. You can. You just pay attention when you do, intentionally noticing the texture, smell, and taste of the ice cream as you eat instead of shoveling it in. Keep in mind that as your mindful eating skills develop you will be able to eat in any circumstance mindfully. It's just a matter of where you put your focus.

DISAPPOINTING FORBIDDEN FOODS

Another "downside" of mindful eating is that you may find that your favorite foods, those forbidden treasures that you typically deny yourself, don't actually taste good. This can be very disappointing. For example, you finally "allow" yourself to have pizza only to discover that it is too greasy for you. Or you bring home a nice warm apple pie only to determine that it is sickeningly sweet. You may feel sad when you learn that your beloved foods are not so wonderful after all. You've been avoiding them for so long and now, when you have "permission" to include them in your diet, they let you down. If this happens to you, give yourself time to grieve their loss. It may seem silly to you to grieve the loss of nachos or fudge brownies, but letting go of these foods is a form of loss and losses need to be grieved. Part of mindful eating is being mindful of your emotions and grief is an emotion that is worthy of your attention. So, mourn the end of your love affair with these former cherished foods and rejoice in the good news that other foods will taste awesome. Experiment and you will find new foods that, when eaten mindfully, are even more satisfying and fulfilling than your former favorites.

Garrett is an excellent example of someone who struggled with disappointment when he discovered that Big Macs no longer taste good to him. A truck driver for most of his adult life, Garret was used to eating on the run. When his wife suggested he learn about mindful eating, he was less than enthusiastic. The idea of taking time to eat and savor his food was totally unappealing. When his doctor told him that his lifestyle (driving eight to ten hours a day and only eating fast food) was hurting him, he acquiesced.

As I do with all my TAME participants, I encouraged him to continue choosing foods that he wants to eat but instead of rushing through his meal, or worse yet, eating while driving, I asked him to take the time to eat whatever he has chosen mindfully and without distractions. For Garret, that meant getting his fast food and then sitting in his truck or inside the restaurant and eating his meal slowly, paying attention to each and every bite. Garrett was pleased that I "did not take away [his] Big Macs" and agreed to eat his "fast food slowly." Every day for the next week, Garrett went to McDonalds and ordered his usual fare—two Big Macs, large fries, apple pie, and a super-sized Coke. And every day, he ate his meal in his truck. No radio. No cellphone. "No nothing."

For the first few days, he couldn't believe his luck. He finally found a "diet expert" who said he could he eat Big Macs. By the fifth day, however, things were starting to change. Garret told his wife he was "getting sick of Big Macs and that they really don't taste so good." In the past, when he ate them quickly, polishing them off with fries and a Coke, he never really tasted them beyond the first bite. Now that he was tasting each bite, the Big Macs were greasy, messy, and bland. He was devastated. Now what was he going to eat? With the encouragement of his wife, his fellow TAME participants and me, Garrett branched out. He tried other kinds of fast foods, including salad bars and pre-made selections in supermarkets.

However, for weeks following the Big Mac experiment, Garett lamented over his beloved hamburgers. What he missed the most was what he thought the Big Macs tasted like. He would say things like, "I thought they tasted good, I really did!" and "How could I be so wrong? They must have changed the recipe." Eventually, Garret found some other favorites, including homemade goodies his wife lovingly prepared, and Big Macs became part of his past.

LESS IS MORE

One more dispiriting observation is that you might discover, as you become a mindful eater, that you need much less food than you thought you did. We, as a culture, are so used to eating large portions of everything that a "normal" portion seems skimpy. As you tune into your body and its needs, you will find that, at times, a smaller amount of food is all you require. Each time you choose to eat in accordance with your body's needs, including eating less, you are moving closer to your goals because eating less is what will help you lose the excess weight that you have been trying to get rid of. If you feel deprived by smaller portions, take heart, you can always eat this food again the next time you are hungry. What at first seems like a disappointment will in the end be liberating and life changing.

In the next chapter, we will begin Step One – Cultivating a Meditation Practice. With the foundation we have laid so far, you are ready to begin. Let's get started.

MINDFUL BITE:

The only way to fail is to not try.

Chapter Four
Step One - Cultivating a Meditation Practice

*Meditation practice isn't about trying to throw ourselves away
and become something better, it's about befriending who we are.*

Ani Pema Chodron

Welcome to Step One. Here you will begin the process of establishing a meditation practice. We will look at what meditation is, why it is valuable, and why it is recommended for mindful eating. I will teach you how to meditate and offer you a script and a schedule to get you started. We will explore tools such as a meditation log, cushions, benches, and timers. We will finish with tips on how to improve your meditation practice.

WHAT IS MEDITATION?

For some people, the thought of meditation conjures up images of long-bearded gurus sitting in the lotus position for hours on end removing themselves from society so they can contemplate the world. Others believe meditation means silencing the mind of all thoughts and feeling calm and peaceful at all times. While there are some gurus with long beards who meditate in solitude, the rest of us mortal beings don't have such a luxury. We meditate as part of our active daily lives. And as for silencing the mind, forget about it! Not only is that extremely difficult—if not nearly impossible—it is not necessary to get the benefits meditation has to offer.

Simply put, meditation is the practice of turning your attention to, and focusing your concentration on, a single focal point such as a sound, an object, an image, a movement, or your breath, for the purpose of increasing your awareness to the present moment.

How you choose your object of awareness varies among different forms of meditation. There are many different types. Some that you may have heard of include Transcendental Meditation, Kundalini Meditation, Qi Gong, Zazen, Mantra Meditation, Movement Meditation, and Mindfulness Meditation. Let's look at each of them.

Transcendental Meditation (TM), made famous by Maharishi, has as its goal enlightenment. A Hindu tradition, TM has the practitioner sitting in a lotus position, silently chanting a mantra, and seeking to rise above the world's negativity.

Kundalini Meditation has its roots in Buddhist and Hindu teachings and focuses on one's breath as it flows through the energy centers of the body, starting with the base of the spine. Using breath, mantras, hand placements and chants, the practitioner seeks awakening and enlightenment. This meditation is often done in yoga classes.

Qi Gong is a form of exercise that has meditative qualities. Begun in China, Qi Gong combines breathing techniques and movement. This form of meditation is very popular because of its health benefits and is often practiced outdoors.

Zazen, or seated meditation, is a tradition from Zen Buddhism and is an unguided form of breathing meditation. To practice Zazen, you sit with a straight back and center your attention on your breathing.

Mantra Meditation uses a single word or sound, such as "Om," as the object of awareness. This word or sound is repeated silently or aloud throughout the practice session as a way to focus the mind.

Rather than focusing on one's breath or a sound or word, Movement Meditation focuses on gentle movement. For example, a gentle swaying or rocking movement can be used. Light stretching or slow walking are also examples of movement meditation. Some beginners prefer movement meditation as a way to start a meditation practice because they find it easier than using their breath.

Lastly, there is Mindfulness Meditation. Also coming from the Buddhist tradition, Mindfulness Meditation uses the breath to explore the workings of the mind and learn to be present. Mindfulness Meditation acknowledges that the mind wanders and rather than trying to shut those thoughts out, the mindfulness practitioner lets the mind wander and accepts whatever thoughts emerge. When these thoughts appear, they are noticed briefly and then attention is redirected to the breath.

WHY MEDITATION IS VALUABLE

Meditation in general, and Mindfulness Meditation in particular, have been shown to have significant therapeutic value, both physically and psychologically. Here's a sample of what mindfulness meditation can do for you:

- Physically:
  - Increase your immune system
  - Decrease pain and inflammation
- Emotionally:
  - Increase emotional regulation
  - Increase positive emotions
  - Increase emotional intelligence
  - Decrease depression, anxiety, and stress
  - Decrease binge eating

- Socially:
  - Increase social connections
  - Increase compassion
  - Decrease loneliness
- Cognitively:
  - Increase focus and attention
  - Increase memory
  - Increase creativity

That's quite a list. We'll go deeper into these benefits in Step Five: Expanding Mindfulness to the Rest of Your Life. Hopefully, what I've listed above is enough to get you more interested in establishing a meditation practice.

WHY MEDITATION IS THE FIRST STEP TO MINDFUL EATING

At this point, you may be wondering why meditation is the first step to mindful eating. I'm sure you were expecting something like keeping a food diary or tossing out your junk food to be first. No, not this time. This time you will begin by going inward, by learning to connect to your body and mind in a way you may have never done before. By going inward, you will be developing the skill of Inner Wisdom which will be discussed in the next step. Being able to focus on what is going on with your body and mind will be very helpful to becoming a mindful eater. This is where meditation comes in. But don't worry, I will not be teaching you to become a navel-gazing sage sitting on a mountaintop. No, the kind of meditation you will be doing is for regular everyday folk who are too busy to pursue enlightenment, like Madeline.

Madeline, a busy oncology doctor with twin six-year-olds, was less than pleased when I explained that the first step to mindful eating is a daily meditation practice. Hardly able to find time to come to the TAME sessions, she was convinced she would never find time to meditate. I understood. I am busy too. We all are. Between seeing clients in my clinical psychology practice, teaching at college and grad schools, and coaching mindful eating, my days are pretty full.

A requirement of my becoming a qualified MB-EAT instructor was having a regular meditation practice. I, too, worried that I would not find the time to devote to meditation, but since I was committed to learning MB-EAT, I found a way. I began with ten minutes in the morning. If I really didn't have the time in the morning, I would steal away ten minutes around lunchtime. If that didn't work, then before I turned off the lights to go to bed, I would do my ten minutes. I did whatever I had to do to get my ten minutes in. Then something interesting started to happen. I noticed that on the days when I spent ten minutes meditating in the morning, I had more time during the day. I noticed that I was becoming more efficient, more focused, and better able to concentrate, so other tasks took less time. I felt as if I were creating time. It is kind of like discovering you have more energy as a result of exercising, even though you had to drag yourself to the gym.

I shared all this with Madeline, and she was intrigued by my remark that I felt as if I were creating time. If meditating could add hours to her day, she was all for it. After a few weeks of finding the time for a short daily practice, Madeline reported that while meditation did not add hours to her day, she felt, as I did, more productive than ever before.

HOW TO MEDITATE

Meditating is not as complicated as people believe. As I have said before, it is not about clearing your mind of all thoughts. It is not about sitting for hours without moving. It's not about a heightened sense of relaxation (although that often comes with it). Nor is it about religion or even spirituality. It is about settling in, focusing your attention, and being quiet for a little while.

We will be using mindfulness-based meditation with the breath as the object of our attention. Your mind will wander and that's okay. With mindfulness meditation, you notice the thoughts that show up, maybe label them with words such as "Thinking," "Complaining," or "Daydreaming" and then direct your attention back to your breath. You will do this over and over again. That's meditating.

In a moment, I will give you a script to guide you in your first meditation. Before I do that, let me describe briefly what will happen.

Here's what a meditation practice looks like.

1 First, you set aside a time for your practice. Choose a time which you will consistently reserve for meditation. Many people find mornings, late afternoons, or early evenings preferable to right before bed to prevent falling asleep. You choose what will work best for you. You may have to try out several times of the day to find your sweet spot, but you will. Please note, if there are other people present when you are ready to practice, ask them not to disturb you. Move pets and children out of the area. That may sound harsh, but this is your time, and it is sacrosanct.

2 Second, you choose a spot for your practice. It can be a corner of a room. A particular chair. A place outdoors. Place a timer or some other device nearby to keep track of time. You don't want to keep checking your watch to see how long you have been going. I address the creation of a special meditation space in a little bit.

3 After you have your time and place selected, you pick your preferred posture: sitting, kneeling, or lying down. If you are not sure, start by sitting in a chair where you can maintain a relaxed, straight back. Some people find sitting cross-legged on a raised pillow comfortable. If you want to lie down, that's fine, just be sure not to get drowsy; you don't want to fall asleep. There are cushions, mats, pillows, and benches available to help you find the position that suits your body best. When I started, I sat in a straight-backed chair with a thick cushion under my feet. Without the cushion, my feet barely touched the floor and I did not feel grounded. Now I sit on the floor using cushions. You can order meditation tools online. Just Google "Meditation Cushions" and see what pops up.

4   Once you have your place and position in order, decide the length of time you would like to practice and set a timer. There are guided meditations available on apps like Insight Timer which you might like. Also, you can use headphones if you are listening to a guided meditation or to block out extraneous noise.

5   Now it is time to meditate.

In the beginning, set a goal to meditate six out of every seven days. Start with five minutes and add more minutes as you are ready. Don't worry, you'll know when to lengthen your practice. I find it effective to keep a meditation log. You might want to keep a log too. In your log, record when you meditated, where, for how long, how it felt, and any other thoughts or comments that you find important.

Please remember that learning to meditate is a skill and it may take a while for you to feel comfortable. If you notice you are judging yourself with thoughts such as: "I'm too distracted"; "I can't stop thinking"; "This is too hard"; or, "I'm too restless," simply observe these thoughts and return your attention back to your breath. In time, this will change. It's all part of the practice.

BEGINNING MINDFULNESS MEDITATION SCRIPT

Here is a script for a five-minute beginning mindfulness meditation. It is derived from Dr. Jean Kristeller's MB-EAT research. Feel free to make a recording of this meditation for your own use.

Before you begin, get comfortable in a chair, sitting with a relaxed but straight posture. If you prefer to lie down, find a position that is comfortable, but not so comfortable that you will become drowsy. Loosen any tight clothing. Allow your hands to rest comfortably in your lap, on your thighs, or by your side, and gently close your eyes.

Allow your body to become still. Allow your shoulders, chest, and stomach to relax. Focus your mind on the feeling of your breathing. Begin by taking two or three deep breaths, letting the air flow all the way into your stomach, without any push or strain, and then flow gently back out again.

Take two or three more deep breaths, noticing an increased sense of calm and relaxation as you breathe in the clean, fresh air, and breathe out any sense of tension or stress.

Now let your breathing find its own natural, comfortable rhythm. Focus your attention on the feeling of your breath as it comes in at the tip of

*your nose, and back out again, letting your stomach rise and fall natu-
rally with each breath.*

*As you continue, you will notice that the mind becomes caught up with
thoughts and feelings. You may notice bodily sensations. You may find
yourself remembering the past, thinking about the future, or fantasizing. This is to be expected. This is the nature of the mind.*

*When you notice this—without self-judgment—simply observe that the
mind is doing this and then return your attention to your breath. Simply
ride with the flow of breath, feeling it move in and out with a gentle,
natural rhythm.*

*If it becomes difficult to not get caught up in thoughts, let your mind
gently count from one to ten with each breath, and then begin again.
When your mind is quieter, you can stop counting and return to the
feeling and experience of the breath. Take two or three more deep
breaths.*

*And now, gently bring your attention back into the space of this room.
Move around gently in your chair or where you are lying. When you
are ready, open your eyes and gently stretch out.*

CREATING A MEDITATION SPACE FOR YOURSELF

In the steps I outlined for you above, I wrote about picking a spot to do your
meditation practice. Something I did for myself that helped me establish a daily
practice was setting up a special space in my home for my meditation sessions. I
chose a corner of my home office near my reading chair. I placed my cushions on
the floor and I kept them there all the time. Seeing them helps me remember to sit
for a few minutes each day. I also have a blanket close by in case I get cold and I have
some water and a timer on a table nearby. My meditation space is nothing fancy or
special, but it is there. You might want to set up such a "sacred" space for yourself.
Here's how:

1 Start with your cushion, mat, or chair—whatever it is you meditate on.
If you need extra bolsters or cushions for support, be sure to include them.

2 Find a location in your home or office that feels good to you. Inviting.
Peaceful. Calm.

3 Place the cushion down and sit. How does it feel to be in this spot? Is
there enough room for you? Do you feel cramped? Exposed? Open? Free?

4 If you like this spot, great! If not, keep searching. In warmer months,
you might want to set up your meditation space outdoors in a garden or on
a patio. In the winter, you might set up near a fireplace or heater. Wherever
you choose, make sure it has a comfortable temperature or have a blanket,

pair of socks, or fan nearby.

5   Also, make sure that the spot you have chosen is relatively quiet. If you live in a city as I do, you might want to pick a spot in the back of your home, away from city traffic and noise. If you have a neighbor whose dog barks a lot, find a spot as far from its howls as possible. It's unlikely that there will never be any noise, but it helps to avoid the obvious ones if you can.

6   Once you have chosen your spot, make it special. Add candles, ornaments, statutes, or whatever else brings you joy. You can decorate it with cards and pictures that are special to you. Because my meditation space is near my reading chair, I am surrounded by books and other items that are meaningful to me. Wherever you choose, make it a sacred space that is used only for your practice and nothing else.

7   Finally, you might want to have a timer, water bottle, or cup of tea on hand. These little extras can make your meditation time more enjoyable.

HOW TO IMPROVE YOUR MEDITATION

Every time I saw my client Peter, he complained to me that he was "meditating wrong."

When I asked him to tell me why he thought that way, he answered, "I can't do it. My mind is constantly filled with random thoughts. I have no control over them."

I listened to what he said and then tried to reassure him by explaining that a person can't meditate wrong, but he wasn't buying it, so I gave him these five tips on how to "improve" his practice. Here they are for you.

5 TIPS TO IMPROVE YOUR MEDITATION PRACTICE:

TIP #1: REMOVE ALL JUDGEMENT

If you are like Peter, you may be coming to the idea of establishing a daily meditation practice with some preconceived notions of what it should look like and how you should feel. You may have certain expectations about yourself, your "performance," and your experience. I encourage you to let all that go. Allow your practice to be whatever it is. Accept that some days will be "good" days (however you define that) and others will be "bad" days. Accept that some practices you will enjoy more, others less. It's all good. If you keep in mind that the essence of mindfulness meditation is increasing your awareness, whenever you do that, you are meditating. It's actually that simple.

TIP #2: SIT EVEN WHEN YOU DON'T FEEL LIKE IT

The key to improving your practice is by practicing. As Nike taught us, "Just Do It!" Or, as a wise mentor of mine once said, "Don't do something, just sit there!" That's my instruction to you. Just sit. Get into the daily habit of sitting on your cushion or chair or mat or floor, turning on your timer or guided recording, and being there. Even if you don't focus on a single breath, sit there. Even if you spend the entire time drafting a memo in your head, sit there. Even if you complain to yourself about meditating, mindful eating or me, sit there. By sitting there when you don't want to, you are training yourself to be present. You are training yourself to not act on your impulses (i.e., get up and walk away). You are developing the discipline to be with yourself and to act on your own behalf. Eventually, you will notice a breath or two. Eventually, your thoughts will still. Eventually, you will be meditating.

TIP #3: LIE DOWN IF THAT HELPS

A dear friend of mine, who has been meditating for many years, told me once that she began her practice lying down. She revealed that she really wanted a meditation practice to help with a chronic health issue but could not get herself to sit in a chair for any length of time. At first, she judged herself, believing that she was being "bad" for not sitting crossed-legged on the floor. When she learned the principles of non-judgment and self-acceptance, she gave herself permission to lie down.

There is nothing "wrong" with lying down. In fact, some meditations, such as the Body Scan Meditation, are done lying down. Happy to know that she was not "bad," my friend did her meditations for years lying down. Then, during a retreat, she sat up and discovered that she could now sit for her practice. If she hadn't given herself permission to lie down, she might never have established her practice in the first place. Now she is sitting every day and enjoying her meditations. If you are having a hard time sitting, I give you permission, if you need it, to lie down.

TIP #4: ADJUST THE LENGTH OF TIME YOU PRACTICE

Adding or subtracting minutes from your practice can make your meditation go smoother. Some people find they get restless after five or ten minutes. If that's you, make your entire session only five or ten minutes. Others find that the first five or ten minutes are the "hardest," but that if they sit for longer, their mind settles down and they can focus on their breath more easily. Extend or contract your practice to suit your needs. Just because I, or another teacher, tell you to do something doesn't mean you have to do it. Make this practice your own. Do it your way.

TIP #5: GO TO MEDITATION CLASSES

My last tip for improving your meditation practice is that you enroll in meditation classes. Meditation centers, continuing education classes, and drop-in sessions are popping up all over as meditation becomes more mainstream. You can even find live online classes. Practicing with others and having a teacher nearby to help is a very effective way to build your skills and stamina. Plus, you might make some new friends! This is the tip Peter took to heart and it worked wonders for him.

Peter and I are fortunate. We live in cities that have a lot of meditation options. Peter did some research online and discovered that his local library was sponsoring meditation classes every Wednesday night. These classes were "drop-in" classes, meaning you didn't need to enroll. All you had to do was show up. Peter admitted to me that he was nervous about going. He was sure he'd be the only man there and the only one who "can't meditate." I encouraged him to give it a try and he agreed to go.

As he approached the meeting room, he noticed there were ten chairs placed in a circle. Four of the chairs were occupied. Scattered around the circle were two women and two men. One of the men was the teacher. He motioned for Peter to join the circle. Peter sat down between one of the women and the other man. The teacher, an experienced mindfulness meditator himself, was warm and welcoming. He introduced himself to Peter and the other class members followed suit. Two more people entered, and the class began.

The teacher gave a brief explanation of mindfulness meditation and then led the group in a thirty-minute practice. When Peter opened his eyes at the conclusion of the meditation, he found it hard to believe that thirty minutes had passed. He was hooked. He continued to attend the library drop-in class every Wednesday night for six months and in the end, the guy who "can't meditate" was meditating every day.

You can too. Begin your practice today. Do what you can and begin again tomorrow. You don't have to be perfect, just practice.

With your meditation practice started, we will move into Step Two and cultivate your Inner Wisdom.

STEP ONE SUMMARY:

The foundation for mindful eating is a daily mindfulness meditation practice. To begin cultivating your meditation practice, meditate five minutes a day as often as you can. Add minutes to your daily practice at a pace that feels right for you. Eventually, try to have a thirty-minute daily practice. You can practice with the guided meditations I provided in this book or with ones you find online, or you can practice in silence using a timer to let you know when you are done. Keep a meditation log to track your progress and observations.

MINDFUL BITE:

Practice meditating a few minutes most days and you will establish a mindfulness meditation practice.

Chapter Five
Step Two – Cultivating Your Inner Wisdom

Don't let the noise of others' opinions drown out your own inner voice.
Steve Jobs [Stanford University Commencement Speech, 2005]

Welcome to Step Two. This step is all about cultivating your Inner Wisdom. Here we will explore the specific elements of Inner Wisdom (hunger, thirst, taste, fullness, and satisfaction), how you develop them, and why using your Inner Wisdom works better than any diet or other outside recommendation.

WHAT IS INNER WISDOM?

Inner Wisdom is best described as using feedback provided by your body to guide you in knowing what is best for you, your health, and your overall well-being. It is information given by your mind and body regarding your hunger, thirst, taste, fullness, and satisfaction. Your body has unique ways of communicating when it is hungry, what to eat or drink, and how much. By developing your Inner Wisdom, you will be able to act in accordance with your body's instructions and foster a relationship with food that is nurturing and sustaining.

There is a guidance system within your body that is home to your Inner Wisdom. It is your Enteric Nervous System (ENS). Located within the esophagus, stomach and intestines, this nervous system is sometimes referred to as the "belly brain." The ENS is responsible for sensing and controlling your digestive tract. This system communicates with your brain to inform you what, when, and how much to eat.

Your digestive system also contains hormones and neurochemicals, including serotonin, dopamine, and norepinephrine. These substances are intricately involved in using food as energy and also experiencing emotions. Have you ever said, "I'm sick to my stomach over that news," or "that makes me want to gag"? This is the "brain in your belly" guiding you.

As you cultivate your Inner Wisdom, you will learn to make sense of the messages you receive and use their information to guide your choices. Your Inner

Wisdom is so powerful that it will help you more than any diet ever could.

INNER WISDOM IS BETTER THAN A DIET

The truth is, if you are looking for a lifetime solution to weight and eating issues, Inner Wisdom is the ticket. Diets are, by their very nature, short-term interventions that rarely live up to their promises. Statistically speaking, anywhere from 65–95% of people regain weight lost by dieting.

A reason why diets don't work for the long-term is that they do not change your relationship to food or cultivate habits that become second nature. Diets are typically offered as a protocol to follow which, while followed, often lead to a drop in weight. Rarely, however, can these protocols be followed indefinitely. Furthermore, diets can be thought of as generalized sources of information that benefit some people but not others. Why is that? Why might a diet that is endorsed by success stories fail for you? And how can experts espouse the benefits of a high-carb diet one day and then the next day other experts renounce that diet and advocate for a low-carb one? My answer is that while often well-intended, diets do not consider a person's unique body chemistry, physiological needs, or psychological makeup. We are not all the same. A one-size-fits-all diet is doomed to fail. What is not doomed to fail is your Inner Wisdom.

Inner Wisdom is your unique, one-size-fits-you path to achievable, maintainable, healthy weight loss. Once you understand your Inner Wisdom and are tuned into it, you will never be lured by the promise of a diet again.

ELEMENTS OF INNER WISDOM: HUNGER, THIRST, TASTE, FULLNESS AND SATISFACTION

It's now time to get to know your Inner Wisdom. Your Inner Wisdom will be your personal guide on your mindful eating journey. By listening to your Inner Wisdom, you will become aware of your body's signals for hunger, thirst, taste, fullness, and satisfaction. As you become familiar with these signals, you will put yourself in a position to make better choices of what, when, and how much to eat. When you heed your Inner Wisdom and make decisions consistent with its advice, you will transform your eating habits and find peace with food. We will explore each element of Inner Wisdom. I will additionally provide you with meditations (including scripts) which you can practice to help you understand what each Inner Wisdom element means and how it shows itself to you. Let's begin with Mindful Hunger.

MINDFUL HUNGER

If mindfulness is about awareness, then Mindful Hunger is about being aware of your hunger—your physical hunger. Physical hunger is different than emotional hunger, which we will explore in great detail in Step Four: Exploring Your Emotions without Overeating. Physical hunger is about being attentive to the sensations in your body that tell you when you are hungry and need nourishment, how hungry you are (meaning how much nourishment you need), how and when your hunger changes as you eat or drink something, and how different foods and beverages affect your hunger in the moment and later on.

So, how do you know when you are physically hungry? When you learn to pay attention, you will "hear" the clues your mind and body send. These clues can be physical or psychological. Here are some examples of the clues that signal hunger.

The physical signs of hunger include dizziness, wooziness, rumbling stomach, jitteriness, queasiness, weakness, headache, throat tightness, lack of concentration, and an empty feeling in the gut.

The psychological signals include irritability, prickliness, moodiness, grumpiness, crabbiness, grouchiness, and a preoccupation with food.

What does hunger feel like for you? Do any of the signs listed above seem familiar? Do the signals vary depending upon how hungry you might be?

Let's look at the following example from my client Karen to see how and when hunger strikes.

It was almost noon on a typical Tuesday in Karen's busy real estate office. She was in the middle of a call with a prospective buyer when she felt a slight grumbling in her stomach. Since she was in the course of setting up a showing for a hard-to-sell condo, she didn't want to get off the phone. Once she did get off the phone, she decided to postpone having lunch so she could get the paperwork arranged for the showing set for later that evening. Halfway through collecting the documents, Karen found herself thinking about the leftovers she packed for lunch. To hear her tell it, "Images of Kung Pao Chicken danced in my head."

No longer able to concentrate on her work, Karen decided to eat. She went to the office kitchen, grabbed her insulated bag from the fridge, poured herself an iced tea, and placed the container of Kung Pao into the microwave. As the container circled inside the oven, Karen noticed herself getting hungrier. Now she was really hungry and was even salivating a bit. The microwave pinged. Karen pulled out her piping hot lunch and sat down to eat. The first few bites were delicious, just the right amount of spice and juicy flavor. After a few more bites, Karen noticed that she started to feel full but kept eating. However, now the food wasn't quite as tasty as before. She finished the container, rinsed it out, grabbed the rest of her iced tea, and returned to her desk.

Karen stared at her computer for a bit, feeling quite full. She found it hard to jump back into preparing for her meeting, so she distracted herself with phone calls and emails. Around 3:00 p.m., a colleague came by and invited Karen for a coffee run. Karen told me that she was still full from lunch but welcomed the interruption, so she went with her friend.

At the café, she ordered her usual afternoon snack—a chai latte and chocolate chip cookie.

While waiting for the latte to be prepared, Karen nibbled on the cookie. "Funny," she told me, "It was chalky and bland. Not at all what I was expecting."

When I asked her what she did with the cookie, she said, "I ate it, duh!"

Does any of this sound familiar? Did you see when Karen's hunger played a role in what and when she ate and when it didn't? Or how Karen being hungry made her food seem tastier and not being hungry changed that?

There are three times to be mindful of your hunger. The first is at the start of a meal or snack. Observing your hunger at this time can help you decide if you want to eat or not.

The second point at which to be mindful is partway through the meal or snack. Sometime after you have been eating, your hunger will subside. Being mindful of when this happens will assist you in determining if you want to continue eating or to stop.

The final time to be mindful of hunger is at the end of your meal or snack. Check in with yourself to see if you have had enough. It is possible to still be hungry at the end if, for example, you did not provide yourself with enough food to eat. If you are still hungry, keep eating until you mindfully decide you are not. If you are not sure, wait about twenty minutes and reassess. If you are hungry then, eat something.

It may be helpful for you to create a Hunger Awareness Scale to capture the true nature of your hunger. If one is "not hungry at all" and ten is "so hungry you'd eat anything," where does your hunger fall when you check into it? Using this type of scale, people report that a four or five level of hunger is the best time to eat.

MINDFUL HUNGER MEDITATION

Below is a meditation script that you can use to guide you in identifying your level of hunger. You can use it at the beginning, middle, and end of your meal or snack. It only takes a minute or two and is very effective.

> Take a moment to center yourself and bring your attention to your breath. If you would like to, you can close your eyes, but you don't have to. You can do this meditation with your eyes in a soft gaze. Breathe in and out several times and then bring your attention to your entire body. Using the Hunger Awareness Scale you created for yourself, notice where on the scale your hunger falls. How do you know? Notice how your body is communicating its hunger to you. When you are ready, bring your awareness back to your breath and then back to the room.

MINDFUL THIRST

The next element of Inner Wisdom is Mindful Thirst. Before we become mindful, we may mistake thirst for hunger and eat instead of drink. As a nation, we are dreadfully dehydrated. According to doctors, as many as 75% of Americans may be dehydrated, meaning they do not have enough water in their bodies for optimal functioning. The question to ask yourself the next time you think you are hungry is, "Could I be thirsty instead?" If you are not sure, drink a glass of water. Wait about ten minutes or so and ask again. Learn the difference between thirst and hunger in your body. Pay attention to how much water is the right amount of water for you. Is it the recommended eight glasses a day or do you need more or less? Do your needs change because of your exercise routine, the weather, or the foods you consume?

I don't remember ever meeting anyone who didn't like to drink water until I met Olga. Olga, a lovely middle-aged woman with a delightful Eastern European accent, made it very clear that she doesn't drink water. When I asked her why not, she shrugged. I turned to the other members of her TAME group for help. Upon inquiry, she admitted that she doesn't like how water tastes. She also said she never got into the habit of drinking water and can't understand why American women carry water bottles with them wherever they go. This remark made the other women in her group laugh.

She was right, many of us do carry water bottles with us. When asked if she ever got thirsty, she replied emphatically, "No!"

The group pressed her about getting thirsty when she exercises, and she said with a smile: "Who exercises?!"

I wasn't so sure about the truth of her remark that she never gets thirsty, so I suggested to Olga that she probably does get thirsty but that she does not recognize the sensation as thirst. I asked the TAME members to tell Olga how they know when they are thirsty. Their answers included: "My lips get dry"; "My throat gets hoarse"; "I get a headache"; "My skin itches"; Olga listened intently and then shrugged again.

I asked Olga if she were willing to do an experiment. I asked her to drink a small glass of water (maybe three or four ounces) before she ate anything. I explained that if she were in fact thirsty rather than hungry, giving herself some water would reduce her need to eat. Eager to let go of fifty pounds, she agreed. I suggested that the other TAME members do the same and notice if having some water before eating made a difference in what and how much they ate.

The following week, Olga came to her TAME meeting carrying a beautifully decorated water bottle. When asked, she said she did the experiment and that several times drinking the water made her not want to eat. She was so happy about that outcome she purchased the water bottle for herself as a gift.

"I feel like an American woman," she exclaimed, raising the bottle over her head in victory.

During Olga's TAME group, clues about how one knows she's thirsty were offered. How do you know if you are thirsty? Do you get a dry mouth? A headache? Pay attention and see how your body lets you know it wants something to drink. Try the experiment I suggested to Olga and drink some water before you eat to see if doing so affects your hunger. If you are not sure if you are hungry, drink a glass of water and wait. If you are hungry, your body will let you know.

MINDFUL TASTE

As an introduction to mindful eating, you did the Raisin Exercise. If you didn't do it when I first presented it, now would be a good time to go back and try it. If you did do it, think back to that experience. Close your eyes and remember bringing the raisin to your lips, placing it in your mouth, and tasting it for the first time. Then remember biting into it, noticing the burst of flavor. Those steps with the raisin were the start to mindful taste.

Without paying deliberate attention to our food, we often eat without tasting. We can feel the food in our mouth, but often it gets swallowed so quickly the tongue barely has a chance to participate. This is especially true if you are a fast eater or a distracted one.

Did you know that a tongue has 2,000 to 8,000 taste buds? These taste buds, or gustatory cells as the scientists call them, can sense five different flavors: salty, sweet, sour, bitter, and savory. How many of those flavors do you taste when you eat? Years ago, I knew a woman who owned a restaurant. She could taste a sample of any dish and describe precisely what ingredients went into it. Now that's tasting!

An extremely enjoyable part of mindful eating is savoring our food. Learning to really taste what we are eating and drinking can lead to greater satisfaction, a desire for less food, and corresponding weight loss. Think of it as becoming a mindful connoisseur—an aficionado of food and drink.

A word of caution though—as you become more mindful of tasting your food, you may discover that you are eating foods you really don't like. That can certainly be true if you based your food choices on a diet regime or other instruction. Let me ask you, how much cottage cheese have you eaten over the years because of some diet you were on? I rest my case.

I'd like to expose you to a Taste Meditation so you can experience savoring. To do this exercise, you will need some chocolate. That's right, chocolate. I recommend you use a brownie or some other form of chocolate cake so you can break it into pieces. If that does not appeal to you, choose your favorite chocolate bar and divide it up, or grab a few small pieces of individual chocolates like Hershey's Kisses. You will need three pieces. When you have assembled the chocolate, you can begin. As before, I have given you the script below. Again, feel free to make a recorded version for yourself if you like. I use a brownie for this exercise, but you can substitute with your preference as your read the script.

TASTE MEDITATION

On a plate or napkin, place three pieces of brownie. Close your eyes and take a few relaxing breaths. Notice your level of physical hunger as we begin. If you use a Hunger Awareness scale, give your hunger a number.

Now open your eyes and look at the brownies in front of you. Choose one piece and pick it up. Look at it carefully. What do you see? Place it in front of your nose. What do you smell? Close your eyes again and place it into your mouth and let it sit on your tongue. What do you taste?

Bite into it. Does the taste change? What do you notice?

Now slowly chew it. Savor each bite. Where in your mouth are you chewing? What are you tasting? Allow yourself to enjoy this bite of brownie as much as possible. When you are ready, swallow it.

After you finish swallowing, are there still tastes in your mouth? What do you notice? With your eyes still closed, take a few deep relaxing breaths. Now open your eyes and pick up another piece of brownie.

Do as you did with the first piece. Examine it, smell it, let it linger on your tongue and then chew it. Is there anything different about this piece of brownie compared to the first? Does it taste the same, better, or worse? Savor it as you did the first piece, noticing the experience as fully as possible.

Are any thoughts or feelings emerging as you eat the brownie pieces? Notice them without judgment. When you are ready, open your eyes.

Now that you have practiced eating two pieces of brownie mindfully, I give you the option to eat a third piece. You might choose to eat the third piece, or you may decide to stop eating. Either way is fine. Observe how you decided to eat more or to stop, being mindful of the reason why you made the choice you made. If you choose to eat the third piece, slowly lead yourself through the experience. Pay attention to how you feel about eating this type of food. Notice if this time around anything is new or different. When you are ready, open your eyes.

We use chocolate in this meditation because chocolate is often a forbidden food for people. Having the experience of mindfully tasting chocolate can help people feel safe around it, knowing that they can eat small amounts without losing control.

Moving forward, practice tasting your food and notice if paying such attention changes your attitude towards certain foods and whether you find yourself naturally eating less.

MINDFUL FULLNESS AND SATISFACTION

Now that you are eating and drinking more mindfully, let's turn our attention to knowing when you are full and satisfied. Specifically, fullness from a physical point of view and satisfaction from a psychological one.

Being physically full means that your body has received the right amount of food it needs from the meal or snack you have eaten. Physical fullness is a feeling of comfort and ease within your body. You may describe it as feeling "whole," "complete," "finished," "safe," "at peace," or "done."

If you are used to overeating on a regular basis, you may think that to feel full means to feel stuffed. With Mindful Fullness, we desire a more neutral, pleasant feeling.

As with Mindful Hunger, you can create a Mindful Fullness Scale. You can rate one as "not full at all" and ten as "really, really full." Find a number on the scale where you are most comfortable. Maybe a five or six. Practice with this scale to learn when your body feels best.

As you become familiar with your physical fullness you may notice that, while you have eaten enough food to fill your belly, you may not, in fact, be satisfied. In other words, you may feel as if you still want more food. This is not unusual.

When you get to the end of a meal and feel as if you still want more to eat, observe what is going in your body and in your mind. Does your mouth want more? Was the food not tasty and you are looking for something else? Some people like to eat something sweet to end a meal. Personally, I like a small piece of mint chewing gum. That hint of sweetness and mint freshens my breath and allows me to move on to my next task, leaving thoughts of food behind.

If you eat quickly or mindlessly, you may miss feeling satisfied. For example, imagine getting to the bottom of a package of M&M's™ and being surprised there are none left. All that remains is the feeling of wanting more.

Perhaps you are unsatisfied because you chose to eat something you really didn't want. In such a case, you may be physically full but psychologically empty. In other words, you are unsatisfied.

How will you know when you are satisfied? Here are some ways others have found:

- They smile as they eat the last morsel, knowing they can have more when they get hungry again.
- They happily leave food on their plate without second thoughts or feelings of disappointment.
- They walk away from the table without wanting more.
- They don't think about food until the next signs of hunger emerge.

To help you become mindfully satisfied, try the following mindful actions:

- Eat your meal or snack without any distractions. That means no TV, computer, book, or phone. Focus your attention on your food.
- Eat slowly. This is especially important if you are a fast eater. I was a fast eater before I became a mindful eater. Part of the reason I ate quickly was because I always had something else I had to get to. When I taught myself to slow down, I enjoyed my food more, felt more satisfied, and still got my work done. Amazing!

- Pay attention to the taste of each bite. Savor your food. Pretend you're a food critic and really taste what is in front of you.
- Choose a food that you really want, not one that you "should" eat, and give yourself permission to eat the food you have chosen.

By mastering Mindful Fullness and Satisfaction you will find that you enjoy your food more than ever before. What a bonus!

A jolly fellow weighing close to 400 pounds, Reid eats a lot of food but never feels satisfied. He can eat an entire pizza and still want more. Reid was a clinical client of mine before signing up to learn mindful eating. He knew he was an emotional eater and was especially interested in learning how to feel satisfied with less food. His goal was to be able to walk away from the table without feeling as if he still wanted more. Reid paid extra attention to the Mindful Fullness and Satisfaction portions of the TAME Your Appetite program. He couldn't believe it was possible to feel full without feeling stuffed, and he really couldn't believe it would be possible to leave food on his plate.

Of the four actions that could enhance Mindful Satisfaction described above, I asked Reid to pick one to concentrate on. He chose to eat without distraction. For Reid, this meant he had to turn off the TV, go into the kitchen, and eat there. "Torture" was the word he used when he responded to this suggestion. The idea of eating without the TV on was scary for him. The TV was his best friend, his constant companion. Whenever he was home the TV was on. He said it kept him company. I understand that. I hear that a lot from clients who live alone. They are afraid to turn off the TV because they are afraid of the silence. The last thing I wanted to do was create more stress and tension for Reid, so I asked him if he would be willing to eat one snack each day for the next week in his kitchen without the TV. All his other meals and snacks he could eat in front of the TV. Just one snack. Reid agreed.

For one week, he ate one snack at his kitchen table. I asked him to serve himself whatever snack he wanted, as much as he wanted, on a plate or in a bowl (not out of the package or carton). Then I asked him to take a few deep breaths before eating his snack. My last instruction to him was that he should eat one bite at a time, really tasting the food he had chosen. Because Reid worked all day, we agreed that his evening snack could be the snack he experimented with.

The following week, Reid returned more excited than I had ever seen him. He told me that he chose to eat his evening ice cream in the kitchen as we had agreed. He described emptying an entire ice cream carton into a bowl to eat it. On the first and second nights, he ate all the ice cream he put into the bowl. On the third night, he had eaten about three-quarters of the ice cream he served himself when he surprised himself with the thought, *I could stop now.* He chose not to stop but made a mental note of the experience. On the fourth night, the same thing happened. For the fifth night he served himself an entire carton again, but this time when he had the thought, *I could stop now,* he stopped. He sat at the table staring into the bowl that still contained ice cream and marveled at what he was doing. He was actually leaving food uneaten. He felt satisfied that he had had enough and didn't need to finish the entire bowl. On the sixth night, it happened again, and now for the second time in his adult life, Reid chose to leave his beloved ice cream uneaten to melt in the bowl. As he watched it melt, he felt a wave of pride swell up in him. For an instant he thought he *might conquer* his food "problem." On the seventh night, he served himself less ice cream. He put about half the carton in the bowl and placed the rest back into the freezer. He sat down at the table and slowly, mindfully savored the ice cream one delicious bite at a time. When he got to the last bite, he felt satisfied and full.

The joy on Reid's face as he told me about his success was priceless. Reid was on his way to becoming a mindful eater.

PUTTING IT ALL TOGETHER – MAKING MINDFUL CHOICES

Part of what makes mindful eating so appealing is that you are encouraged to choose food you want to eat. In the past, you may have made food choices pursuant to some diet or other form of instruction and became accustomed to choosing a food because it is "allowed," "legal," or "approved." The problem with choosing food this way is that doing so has the potential to disconnect you from your body and its true needs. This could lead you to eat food you may not truly desire, which could result in bingeing later on the food you really wanted. Mindful eating, especially making mindful choices, can prevent that possibility.

This brings us to the last piece of Inner Wisdom, Mindful Choices. Mindful Choices pull together the other parts of Inner Wisdom and guides you to choosing what and how much to feed your body. Once you master this, you will find your relationship with food shifting and mindful eating becoming easier and more rewarding than you could imagine.

In deciding what food or beverage to choose you will take two steps. First, get quiet and ask yourself what you want to eat or drink. Second, imagine how that food or drink will taste and what it will feel like in your body. Not sure how this will work? Okay, try this:

For a moment, picture a turkey sandwich. Can you see it in your mind's eye? The crusty sourdough bread stacked with lettuce and tomato. Spread some mustard or mayo on it if you like. Envision it exactly as you would want it to be. Is your mouth watering? Good, that means your imagination is working! Now, imagine how your sandwich might taste. Is it to your liking? Is there something about it you would want to change? Maybe some cheese or a slice or two of crispy bacon? Or maybe a Kaiser roll would work better than the bread. Now imagine taking a bite of the sandwich and chewing it. Are you enjoying it? Does it taste good? Now swallow your bite. How does

your body respond? Does it feel good going down? Are you getting full?
Is the sandwich satisfying? Are you still hungry? If so, for what? More
of the sandwich? Something else?

This little guided visualization is a handy tool to help you make mindful choices.

Here are some questions you can ask yourself to steer you to the right choice:

1   How hungry am I?

    a. Do I need a lot of food?
    b. Do I need just a snack?
    c. Am I thirsty?

2   What would taste good to me now?

    a. Sweet or sour?
    b. Salty or bitter?
    c. Crunchy or smooth?
    d. Hot or cold?
    e. Spicy or savory?
    f. Do I want to chew or sip?
    g. Do I want to use a fork or my fingers?

3   How would this particular food feel in my mouth?

    a. Smooth?
    b. Prickly?
    c. Pleasant?

4   How would this particular food feel in my stomach?

    a. Pleasant?
    b. Agitating?
    c. Stuffed?
    d. Soothing?

5   How might I feel after I eat this particular food?

    a. Satisfied?
    b. Unsatisfied?
    c. Still hungry?
    d. Too full?

Your answers will change each time you ask them because your body changes. It will need different foods at different times. Be open to what your body prefers. Keep in mind that your body may guide you to food choices which may be different than your usual go-to choices. Such a departure is okay. Allow yourself to become more particular, even picky, about what you eat. Broaden your scope of "acceptable" food choices. Life can become more fun when you vary your diet!

My client Amanda described going to a restaurant with her husband after learning about mindful eating. Here's what happened.

In anticipation of her anniversary dinner, Amanda requested a private session with me. Earlier in the week, her *TAME Your Appetite* group had spent time talking about mindful choosing. During the group, Amanda became painfully aware that she rarely chose what she wanted from a menu because she felt "chained by" her diet food lists. It was now her wedding anniversary and her husband made reservations at a new Italian place they wanted to try. Amanda loves Italian food, especially pasta, but typically avoids it because she is afraid "pasta will make me fat."

In our session, Amanda and I reviewed the Mindful Choice Questions from above. I encouraged her to try making mindful choices, rather than blindly ordering grilled chicken and steamed vegetables as she was known to do. Timidly, Amanda agreed to try and left to meet her husband.

Before opening the menu, Amanda asked herself the mindful choice questions and discovered that she (1) was hungry, (2) was hungry for a full meal, (3) was in the mood for something savory, and (4) wanted to use a fork and knife. Then she opened the menu to review it. She scanned the items and briefly imagined what each would taste like. Her eyes lingered over the Linguine in Clam Sauce. She felt a twinge of guilt at considering such a "fattening" item but, instead of making her decision based on that thought, she checked in with her body. She imagined how that dish would feel if she ate it. A slight smile curled on her face. She knew that the Linguine in Clam Sauce would be the right choice. She asked herself if she wanted anything else. Soup? Salad? Bread? Each time the answer was a clear no. Wine? "Yes, a glass of Chianti would be nice." She placed her order and relaxed into her anniversary celebration.

Not only was she able to make mindful selections, but she also practiced mindful eating throughout the meal. Periodically, she checked in with her hunger, fullness, and satisfaction. She ended up eating only about two-thirds of the entrée. It surprised her that she was able to leave some of the linguini on the plate. In the past, if she "indulged in pasta," she would have "scarfed down the whole thing" because it is not a dish she usually "lets herself have." She and her husband ended the meal with a shared tiramisu, of which Amanda says she had "four scrumptious bites" and left the restaurant feeling happy and proud. What a great anniversary!

Amanda's experience can be yours too with a little bit of practice. Go for it!

A WORD ABOUT CRAVINGS

Over the years, people have complained to me about overwhelming cravings that interfered with any diet they attempted. Cravings are real experiences that can be handled with mindfulness. The important thing to know about cravings is that they will pass; you don't have to give into them. To manage cravings mindfully, try the following:

Recognize if you are physically hungry. If you are hungry, decide what you are hungry for and eat. If what you are hungry for is what you are craving, enjoy a portion of it mindfully.

If you are not physically hungry, assess if you are emotionally hungry. If you are, address your emotional need. Step Four will teach you how to do that.

STEP TWO SUMMARY:

Cultivating your Inner Wisdom is essential for mastering mindful eating. Step Two taught you how to identify your hunger, thirst, taste, fullness, and satisfaction—the key elements for mindful eating. You were also shown how to put them all together to make Mindful Choices. Connecting with your Inner Wisdom in a meaningful way takes time and practice. Use the Mindful Hunger and Fullness Scales you created as often as possible. Practice the Mindful Hunger Meditation once a day or more as desired. Moving forward, continue with your daily mindfulness meditation practice, adding minutes as you are ready.

MINDFUL BITE:

No one knows better than you what is right for your body.

Chapter Six

Step Three – Balancing Your Eating with Outer Guidance

Eat food, not too much, mostly plants.

Michael Pollan

Welcome to Step Three. In this step, you will become acquainted with your Outer Guidance. As the name suggests, Outer Guidance is information you receive outside yourself (as opposed to Inner Wisdom, which comes from within). This guidance will inform your decisions on what, where, when, and how much to eat. Unlike going on a diet, Outer Guidance imparts sound nutritional advice which you can use as you choose. Examples of Outer Guidance are calories, points, portion sizes, nutritional information, and clean eating. You will learn to use this type of information as a way to make the best decisions without following strict rules or admonitions. We will explore how you discover the best Outer Guidance for your unique needs, and I will share one of my client's successful experiences of identifying and employing Outer Guidance.

WHAT IS OUTER GUIDANCE?

When I talk about Outer Guidance, I am talking about reliable, valuable information about the nutritional content and health implications of food. Such information comes from renowned medical and scientific authorities and not from the latest diet guru. You will use such information as a tool to guide your choices in a mindful way. This doesn't mean you will never eat a hot fudge sundae again or that it is necessary to only eat green vegetables and tofu. Not at all. Utilizing Outer Guidance means that you acquire an education about the foods you eat and then make informed choices.

Cultivating Outer Guidance is different than "going on a diet" because you will not be following a prescribed set of rules. Instead, you will decide for yourself which foods, in which quantities, serve your needs best. Diets are typically "one-size-fits-all." Such an approach does not consider each person's unique dietary needs, nor does it take into account that those needs fluctuate day by day, sometimes hour by hour. Only you know what you need, and Outer Guidance helps you figure out which foods work best for you. By cultivating Outer Guidance, you can give up diets forever. Instead, you will develop your own approach to food based on your unique requirements.

WHAT FORMS OF OUTER GUIDANCE WILL HELP YOU MOST?

Finding the right kind of Outer Guidance can seem overwhelming and confusing at first. There is so much nutritional and health advice available you may wonder where to start and what to believe. I have felt that way too. I have had an interest in health and nutrition for a long time and I have read a lot of books and articles on those topics. One way to develop Outer Guidance is to do what I did and start reading, experimenting, and listening to your body. It will tell you what advice is good for you and which you should reject. Let me give you an example from one of my clients.

Valerie loves animals. Her house is full of them: cats, dogs, birds, lizards. The list goes on. Because of her love of animals, Valerie was interested in becoming a vegan. A vegan is a person who eats no animal products at all. She read up on veganism and decided to give it a try. I supported her in her efforts and asked her to keep a journal of what she ate and how her body reacted to her choices.

At first, she was delighted with becoming vegan. She loved all the beans, rice, pastas, and potatoes. She started growing her own herbs and shopping at the farmer's market. She even got herself a juicer to make fresh juice. The first few months went well until Valerie noticed that she was feeling sluggish in the afternoons and her pants were getting tight. She was practicing mindful hunger and mindful fullness, so we were sure she wasn't overeating. The problem was the selection of foods that made up her vegan diet were heavy on the carbohydrates. Valerie discovered that her body wasn't enjoying a diet so rich in starch.

She experimented by adding back in some lean animal protein at each meal and noticed she was feeling more energetic during the day and, while her pants were still tight, they were not getting tighter. She made another adjustment and added protein to her snacks too. Within several weeks, her energy was up, and her pant size was down.

As much as she wanted to be a vegan, Valerie discovered that her body did not. Her body needed some animal protein to function at its best. So, Valerie compromised. She honored her values regarding animals without becoming a vegan by choosing to purchase only cruelty-free protein products. By combining her Inner Wisdom (Mindful Hunger and Mindful Fullness) with the Outer Guidance she got from learning about veganism, Valerie created a relationship with food that suits her perfectly.

You may not want to be a vegan, but you might be interested in heart-healthy dining, clean eating, or anti-aging science. Whatever you are interested in, become a student and learn what you can. Apply your newly gained knowledge to your eating habits and study the results. Keep what works for you and discard the rest.

If studying nutrition is unappealing to you, there is another way to start cultivating your Outer Guidance. You can begin by simply learning the caloric value of food. Using calories (or Points if you are a Weight Watchers veteran) is a simple way to learn the differences among different foods. But let's be clear; I am not advocating you start counting calories (or Points.) Rather, I am suggesting you use calories (or Points) as a way to pick among equally appealing food choices.

Let's say you enjoy both coleslaw and potato salad with your sandwich. The portion of coleslaw you have available to you has 200 calories and the potato salad has 275 calories. If both choices would satisfy you, you could use the calorie differential as a deciding factor and pick the coleslaw to save some calories without any sense of deprivation.

If you participate in my complete 12 Session *TAME Your Appetite* program, we will do something known as the 500-Calorie Challenge. In the Challenge, you intentionally look for ways to reduce your daily intake by 500 calories without feeling deprived. A 500-calorie deficit can facilitate weight loss if that is your goal.

In this step, however, you do not need to intentionally cut out 500 calories. All you need to do is use calories as a way to decide between equally desirable options as a way of practicing Outer Guidance.

WHERE TO FIND OUTER GUIDANCE

Gathering Outer Guidance is not as difficult as you might think. There are books, magazines, blogs, webinars, online courses, Meetups, you name it, for all sorts of nutritional and health-related topics. Keep on the lookout for material about health and wellness (not weight loss) as you gather knowledge that will serve your interests. Learn the benefits of whole unprocessed foods. Visit farmer's markets. Talk to the vendors. Ask questions about their produce and other products.

Another fun way to gain Outer Guidance is to take cooking lessons. Sign up for a lesson in your favorite cuisine and approach the class with mindfulness. Pay close attention to what the chef is doing and how she is doing it. Use all your senses and appreciate every ingredient that goes into the dish.

Whatever way you choose to acquire Outer Guidance, do so with a spirit of playfulness and joy. Outer Guidance is not meant to be a set of stringent rules. It is intended to be information which you will use to nourish your body and nurture your soul.

Let me give you an example from my own life.

At the age of eighty, my late mother was diagnosed with Age-Related

Macular Degeneration (AMD). AMD is an eye disease where those afflicted lose their central vision. For someone who loved to read, knit, and watch TV, this news was devastating. In the years that followed, my mother lost her central vision. She was not totally blind, but the quality of her life had dramatically diminished. It turns out the AMD runs in families and fair-eyed people are especially at risk.

Because of my mother's condition and the fact that I am a fair-complexioned blue-eyed redhead, my optometrist began scanning my eyes on an annual basis for signs of AMD. With this disease, the earlier one detects it, the better the prognosis. In the summer before I turned fifty-seven, my optometrist noticed some very early signs. She told me not to worry and handed me a bottle of supplements designed to facilitate macular health. I did not worry, but I did get busy.

I began reading about AMD and learned that nutrition can play a big role in preventing and/or delaying its onset. I was now in search of Outer Guidance to help me learn which foods are best for me and which I might choose to stay away from. My research led me to a book called, *Macular Degeneration: The Complete Guide to Saving and Maximizing your Sight* by Lylas Mogk, MD, which outlined two dietary recommendations.

They are:

1 Eat lots of dark green leafy vegetables, such as kale, spinach, mustard greens, and broccoli.

2 Use healthy oils (olive, canola, flaxseed, fish) in place of vegetable oils and margarines.

I now use those recommendations to guide my food choices. They are not rigid rules. They are factors I take into account as I go about my life. This is one way I use Outer Guidance as part of my mindful eating practice.

Other authors whose works I have studied include Andrew Weil, M.D. (*8 Weeks to Optimum Health*), Joel Furhman, M.D. (*Eat to Live*), Raymond Francis, M.Sc. (*Never Be Sick Again*) and Tosca Reno, B.Sc. (*The Eat-Clean Diet*). You might find what they have to say enlightening and useful as Outer Guidance for your mindful eating journey.

STEP THREE SUMMARY:

When you collect Outer Guidance and discover what works best for your body, you are creating your own personal guidelines for health and wellness. No commercial diet can do that for you. That is the benefit of Outer Guidance.

Do some research. Read blogs, books, and magazines to assemble the components of your Outer Guidance. Attend lectures, cooking classes, and farmer's markets to broaden your knowledge base. Then begin applying what you learn and assess how your body responds. Keep what feels good and leave the rest. You are in charge. You get to decide how and what to eat.

Or, if research is not your thing, investigate the calories of what you eat.

Decide where you can reduce portion sizes or choose a lower calorie food without compromising on satisfaction. If you want to, simply start cutting down the amount of food you eat while being mindful that this is not a diet and you do not want to feel deprived.

> ## MINDFUL BITE:
>
> **Use Outer Guidance to inform your choices,
> not make them for you.**

Chapter Seven

Step Four - Exploring Your Emotions without Overeating

The best and most beautiful things in the world cannot be seen or even touched. They must be felt with the heart."

Helen Keller

You have arrived at Step Four. Congratulations! By now, you are well on your way to being a mindful eater. I hope you are enjoying the journey. In this Step, we will tackle a topic that is frequently the downfall of many dieters—emotional eating. In this Step, you will learn how to use mindfulness to heal your emotional eating. You will discover ways to be with your emotions without using food as a crutch. The key question you will focus on is: *What are you really hungry for?* In answering this question, you will become aware of different emotions (i.e., Anger, Anxiety, Sadness, and Stress) and how to respond to them in a healthier way. Once again, we will use meditation as the foundation. You will be introduced to other mindfulness-based tools, such as mindful writing. And if you are in need of deeper work, I will point you in the right direction.

WHAT ARE YOU REALLY HUNGRY FOR?

Eating in response to emotions is commonplace. We all do it. The occasional dip into a pint of ice cream after a heartbreak is not a reason for concern. We need to be concerned when turning to food is our habit—when it has become our primary method for coping with our emotions. As I often say, it is what you do most of the time that matters.

I won't go into the details of why we turn to food as a coping mechanism in this book. You can learn more about that in my previous books, especially, *The Best Diet Begins in Your Mind: Eliminate the Eight Emotional Obstacles to Permanent Weight Loss.* Our interest now is recognizing when we are emotionally hungry and what to do about it in a mindful way.

Mindfulness is particularly helpful in distinguishing between physical and emotional hunger. By applying what you know already about Mindful Hunger and Mindful Fullness, you have a good idea of when your body needs food. Any other time you want to eat but do not have the physical signals to do so, you are emotionally hungry.

When you identify that you want to eat something but that your body is not communicating that desire to you, ask yourself, "What am I really hungry for?" and then listen for the answer. Just like you learned to "hear" your body's signals for hunger and fullness, you can learn to "hear" your emotional pain and identify your path to relief. Your path might include calling a friend, taking a walk, having a good cry, soaking in the tub, getting some exercise, or napping. The path to relief may change day to day, or emotion to emotion. If you pay attention, you will know what to do and meditation can help.

Grace was worried about her ability to stop overeating, especially with family. Grace, a thirty-six-year-old woman of Greek descent, comes from a tight-knit family who eats all Sunday dinners and holiday meals together. To hear Grace describe it, every meal is a "Mediterranean feast." I can only imagine how fabulous the food is. I explained to Grace that there are times when we all overeat, offering Thanksgiving, Christmas, and Easter as examples. And, I continued, there are other times when we find ourselves overeating despite our best intentions, citing her family get-togethers. It is at those times where being mindful can be most helpful.

Ending overeating, even in the company of family, is a skill that can be learned. I asked Grace why she thought she overate when with family.

She replied, "It is expected. Everyone indulges, so if I don't it will be noticed."

When I asked if there could be another reason, she shook her head no.

"That's why," she told me.

I went on to explain to Grace that when we overeat, we do so for very important reasons. The excess food or increased eating serves a purpose. Mindfulness can help her figure out what that purpose might be.

I asked Grace to ask herself a simple question at next Sunday's family dinner. I instructed that when she notices she is overeating to ask herself, "What am I really hungry for?" and then listen for the answer. If no answer immediately surfaces, I suggested she step away from the table for a few moments and find a comfortable place to sit where she can do a short meditation. In a relaxed state, she should ask herself the question again and wait for any thoughts or feelings that arise. If after a few minutes nothing happens, that's fine. She can stop the meditation and rejoin her family. Later, she can try the meditation again. Eventually an answer will emerge. Grace said she would try this meditation at her next family meal.

When Grace returned the following week, I asked if she did the meditation and what, if anything, she uncovered.

She shared that when she did the meditation the only thought she had was, *I love the food. It tastes so good. It reminds me of my childhood outside of Athens.*

I followed up by asking her, "Do you miss Greece?"

Grace got silent. Her eyes began to well with tears. Softly, she nodded her head.

"Is it possible you are eating extra food to remain close to your homeland?" I asked. Grace nodded again.

"That's understandable," I assured her, "but," I continued, "if you want to get your weight under control, we will need to find another way for you to feel close to Greece."

We tossed around a few ideas until Grace settled on weekly Skype calls with her favorite cousin who still lives in Athens. In the weeks and months that followed, Grace noticed that she ate less during family dinners on the weeks she spoke with her cousin. By mindfully making the connection between missing her childhood home and the excess eating, Grace became better able to eat according to her Inner Wisdom rather than her emotional pain.

USING MEDITATION TO HELP END EMOTIONAL EATING

You have been using meditation as the foundation for your mindful eating journey since Step One. Now we will explore how meditation can assist you in reducing your emotional eating. The research upon which my *TAME Your Appetite* programs are based provides evidence that mindfulness and mindfulness meditation reduce binge-eating episodes and emotional overeating. In essence, mindfulness helps you to manage your emotions so that you can think more clearly and make better decisions. You are able to respond to an emotional situation rather than react out of habit.

Freedom from emotional eating will come as you change your need to avoid what you are feeling. As you develop the ability to be present with whatever is occurring without needing to act on it, you will let go of using food as a coping mechanism. This new skill coupled with other forms of emotional nourishment will demonstrate to you that you can handle your emotions without food and that you are able to provide yourself with what you need.

Before I introduce you to the meditation for ending emotional eating, let's take a moment to explore your emotions.

WHAT ARE YOU FEELING?

The first step in responding to an emotion is recognizing when you are experiencing the emotion and what it is. This may sound silly to you. How can someone not know what or when they are feeling something? But the truth is, many people are so cut off from their emotions they do not know what they feel. Being cut off from one's emotions can happen when a person (1) has avoided emotions most of their life; (2) only knows how to feel one kind of emotion—usually anger; or (3) they are afraid of their emotions; so, when an emotion arises, they eat to quell it.

Among the most common emotions that people feel are anger, anxiety, sadness, and stress. Meditation is useful for identifying these emotions as well as managing them. In the next chapter, I show you how meditation reduces anxiety, depression, and stress. For now, let's continue to explore what you can do to manage your emotions. We'll use anger as an example.

Anger can be an uncomfortable emotion. When people feel anger, they often fear it and want it to go away. Or they act on it in aggressive ways that cause harm to themselves and others. There is a better way—a mindful way.

Because anger can cause physical discomfort, recognizing its physical sensations is a good starting point for knowing when you are angry. Which physical signs would help you spot your anger? This list may help.

If you are angry, you may:
- Feel hot
- Sweat
- Grind your teeth
- Tighten your jaw
- Clench your fist
- Have a headache or stomachache
- Shake
- Get dizzy
- Experience a rapid heartbeat
- Pace
- Yell
- Cry
- Hit something

Another way to know you are angry is by what is going on psychologically for you.

Here are some signs. Are you:
- Irritable?
- Resentful?
- Verbally lashing out?
- Abrupt?
- Sarcastic?

What thoughts are you thinking?
- Hate?
- Disgust?
- Revenge?
- Harm to self or others?

When you recognize these physical sensations or psychological signs as anger, the next step is acknowledging it. It is one thing to recognize anger, it is another thing to admit that the anger is going on and needs to be felt. Acknowledging it is not the same thing as acting on it. Acknowledging it means not avoiding it, distancing ourselves from it, or finding a way to make it go away. Acknowledging means conceding that it is present, whether you want it or not.

When we are angry, we might want to lash out. We might want to hurt the person who has made us mad. Or anger might make us so uncomfortable that we would do anything to make it go away (i.e., eat, sleep, self-harm). To acknowledge anger means to stay with it, and to allow it to be present even though it might feel bad. To acknowledge other emotions means the same, to admit they are present.

Acknowledgment brings us to acceptance. Acceptance is the willingness to be with the emotion without trying to change or avoid it; to observe it, to explore it. With acceptance you can experience your anger fully, noting the thoughts and physical sensations that accompany it. The more fully you can experience it, the less frightening it will become. You can be present with your anger. Being with your anger makes it a familiar state, one from which you no longer need to escape.

Furthermore, acceptance leads to finding the message or lesson hidden within the emotion. Emotions such as anger have a lot to tell us about ourselves, our lives, and the direction we are going. Just like physical pain is the body's way of telling us something is wrong, emotional pain has a similar message. Through meditation you can hear these messages. By watching what is happening within you and not reacting, you receive the wisdom your emotions want to convey. As the mind calms, you create space for these revelations. Listen for them.

With mindfulness, you allow the thoughts and feelings that are the foundation of your emotions to arise uninterrupted. You create the mental space for reflection and contemplation which allows for new, healthier, more appropriate responses to emerge. In other words, you stop reacting mindlessly and reflexively. Mindfulness allows for a more thoughtful decision about an approach you could take, which serves you better and leads to the result you seek. In the case of anger, you find a more effective retort than losing your cool.

The more you practice mindfulness and mindfulness meditation, the easier it will become to disrupt your ordinary emotional responses. In time, automatically reaching for food when you are emotionally uncomfortable will subside and your emotional eating habit will go away.

To facilitate this happening, use the meditation below to develop the skill of staying with an emotion. You can also use it to address emotional eating whenever you feel it coming on.

MEDITATION FOR ENDING EMOTIONAL EATING

Here is the meditation to help deal with emotional eating. This meditation teaches you to stay present with any emotion. Practice it often so you become comfortable with your feelings. As with any meditation, begin by finding a comfortable position. Loosen any tight clothing. If you want to, close your eyes. If not, lower them slightly and softly gaze at a spot in front of you. You are now ready to begin.

Take several slow, deep breaths. Allow your breath to fill up your lungs and flow into your belly and then gently back out again. Repeat these breaths several more times. Notice if you feel any tension or discomfort in your body. If you do, focus on those areas, silently instructing them to relax.

Continue breathing, allowing your breath to follow its own natural rhythm and depth. Follow the breath in through your nose and out through your mouth. In and out. In and out.

If your mind fills with thoughts, notice them, and then let them go, returning your attention to your breath. Repeat this whenever your mind becomes filled with thoughts. Notice, let go, breathe.

Now, I want you to shift your attention to a specific emotion you are feeling right now or one you want to work with. Allow that feeling to emerge. At any time, if the emotion feels overwhelming, return your attention back to the breath. Stay with the breath until you feel ready to resume the meditation or gently end the meditation.

Then become aware of how this emotion feels in your body. Identify any physical sensations that may be occurring. Place your attention onto to those sensations and label them. For example, "tingling," "aching," "hollowness," or "heaviness." Spend some time with these sensations. Allow them to be. Be curious about them. How might you describe them? What color might they be? What shape? Do they make a sound? Stay with these sensations until you feel at ease with them. When you are ready, take a few deep breaths and notice what thoughts are associated with the emotion.

Are there any words or phrases attached to the emotion? Notice them. Be curious as to why these words or phrases are present. Place your attention on these words and notice how they affect what you feel. Are the words loud and harsh? Are they soft and menacing? What words would comfort you now? Find a word that would soothe you. Focus your attention on that word. Repeat the word several times as you breathe in and out, in and out. Allow that word to be the focus of your meditation for the next few moments. If your mind wanders, simply bring it back to your word.

When you are ready, focus your attention back to just your breath. If any physical sensations have returned, breathe into them and let them go. Continue to focus on your breaths, breathing in calmness, peace, and relaxation, and breathing out any tension, pain, or emotional distress that you may still be holding.

Now become aware of yourself in your room. Begin to visualize the

*room around you. Move your body gently and then when you are
ready, mindfully open your eyes.*

WHAT ARE YOU REALLY HUNGRY FOR?

Becoming comfortable with your emotions is an essential part of mindful
eating and making peace with food. But I would be remiss if I suggested that becoming comfortable was all it took to end emotional eating. Yes, you need to be familiar
and comfortable with your emotions, but you also need to address what the emotional eating is masking. We eat when we don't want to feel something or don't want
to deal with an event or person. Why not?

Above, you learned that emotions have messages in them. What messages
are you hearing? What is it you really need to do, say, or feel to get through whatever is driving your desire to eat when you are not physically hungry? I won't dive
too deep here because my other books can really help with this issue. If you want to
delve into your emotional eating with greater depth, check them out. They are both
excellent self-help books for ending emotional eating. They are listed under Additional Resources at the end of this book.

From now on, whenever you want to eat when you are not hungry, ask yourself the question: *What am I really hungry for?* Listen for the answer. Then, act on
the answer. For example, for the umpteenth time, you had to stay late at work. You
are sick of being asked to do extra work when others get to go home on time. But
instead of standing up for yourself, you acquiesce and stay late. To get through the
extra work, you raid the vending machines. You are not physically hungry for those
processed snacks, so what are you hungry for? Recognition? Overtime pay? The
right to go home on time? Equal treatment? When you know what you are really
hungry for, you can go after it. In this example, maybe you wouldn't mind the extra
work if you could get extra pay. So, what do you do? You build your assertiveness
skills and when you are ready, you ask your employer for more money. Addressing
the real issue is the way out of emotional eating, and the mindful eating skills you
are learning here can help you do just that.

There is another mindful skill I want to introduce to you to help you cope with
your emotions without turning to food. It's called "Riding the Wave of Emotions."

HANDLING EMOTIONS – RIDE THE WAVE

I have spent most of my adult life living in Southern California, and one of
the most beautiful parts of SoCal is the ocean. I have spent countless hours walking
on the beach admiring the view and being entertained by the paddle boarders and
surfers. I love to watch them on the water. The way they balance themselves on the
waves is remarkable. And when they stumble, they get right back up. What a wonderful metaphor for life and for dealing with emotions.

Imagine for a moment that you are standing at the edge of a lake or ocean.

Notice the movement of the water. See how the waves tumble onto the sand and then withdraw. Now imagine that you are in a sailboat. Feel the waves as they carry the boat. Allow yourself to drift with the movement of the waves—peaceful, calm, and soothing.

You can experience emotions the same way, as waves that rise and fall. When you observe your emotions objectively, you can see their natural rhythm. They come on, build up, and then recede. With mindfulness, you can be with your emotions without acting on them, just noticing their ebbs and flows.

To "Ride the Wave," begin by paying attention to where you physically feel the emotion in your body. Observe any sensations present. Is your stomach churning? Are your hands sweating? Do you have a headache? Allow the sensations to rise and fall. Go along for the ride. Do not judge the sensations or try to make them go away. Be curious about them. Witness them without interference.

Next, watch the thoughts that show up. What words or phrases accompany the emotion? Again, do not attach to the thoughts, just notice them. Use your meditation skills to be a curious, impartial spectator of your emotional life. Contrary to what you might think, staying with your emotions, rather than avoiding or denying them, causes them to move along more quickly. Evaded emotions linger. They show up again and again in different ways and at different times. Ride the waves of your emotions and then after they've passed, acknowledge yourself for not eating over them. That's what Jackson did.

At age thirty-eight and 5'10" tall, Jackson isn't extremely overweight but his relationship with food is troubling. Jackson is a binge eater. Whenever he is upset about anything, he heads to the nearest drive-thru and picks up enough food for four people. He drives to the closest parking lot, parks the car, and eats everything he bought. Ashamed of what he did, he tosses the trash into the nearest dumpster before heading home. Waiting for him at home is his beloved wife, Sara.

Jackson and Sara have been married for two years. They met at a surf camp where Jackson was an instructor and Sara was his student. Sara had gone to the class as part of an assignment she got from me. I was working with Sara on her emotional eating and encouraged her to try an activity that challenged her perception of herself. Quite heavy at the time, Sara couldn't imagine herself on a surfboard. With a little encouragement from me, she signed up for "Surf Camp."

As Sara's relationship with food changed and her weight went down, Jackson became interested in what she was doing. At Sara's suggestion, he signed up for one of my *TAME Your Appetite* programs and agreed to try becoming a mindful eater. He was all for meditating and paying attention to his hunger and fullness signals, but when I mentioned emotions, he shut down. That was until I introduced the idea of emotions as waves. Now I had piqued his interest.

Because he is a surfer, Jackson could explain to the other program participants about waves and how, as a surfer, he aims to "be one with the water." The first week after introducing the riding the waves idea, I asked Jackson to practice being with an emotion when he was on his surfboard. Initially put off by my suggestion, he reluctantly agreed. The following Saturday morning, he sat on his board and imagined an argument he had with his brother the night before. As the angry sensations and thoughts swelled, he stood up on the board and he rode the waves. As the waves carried him, he imagined his anger being carried too. As the waves flattened out, so did the feelings.

The next week, Jackson came back to the program session excited to tell everyone about his "angry surfing" and how he was "at one with his anger." This experience gave Jackson the confidence to practice being with his emotions whenever they arose. The more he practiced, the less trips to the drive-throughs he made.

Unless you are a surfer, it is unlikely you will be able to experience your emotions on a surfboard, but you can follow Jackson's lead and "be at one with your anger" on dry land.

MINDFUL WRITING

Earlier, when I made suggestions on how to use this book, I recommended you start a journal to record your journey. If you have done so, you may have noticed how writing is an excellent tool for growth and insight. It is also an excellent tool for coping with emotions. Writing centers us and draws our attention to the moment. It is hard to write and have our focus elsewhere. Writing is a marvelous mindful tool.

About twenty-five years ago, a book titled, *The Artist's Way* by Julia Cameron became a worldwide phenomenon. In her book, Ms. Cameron taught her readers to do "Morning Pages." These were "stream of consciousness" writing sessions done every morning. These sessions were designed to help the reader put thoughts and feeling onto paper without editing. "Morning pages" caught on and soon groups were springing up everywhere in support of this ritual. I recommend "Morning pages" to my clients too. I suggest they take time every morning to write out a page or two of whatever is on their mind. They don't have to worry about spelling or grammar. They don't need to show it to anyone or even read it themselves. Just write. The cumulative effect of these sessions is astounding. Emotions come into focus. Solutions show up. Relief is experienced. Try "Morning Pages" yourself. Try it for a week and see what happens. If you are like some of my clients, "Morning Pages" will become a daily ritual for years on end.

If you don't want to write every morning, write when you feel like it. Write when you are stuck. Write when you can't access your emotions. Write when your emotions feel huge. Use writing as a tool for being with your emotions in whatever way helps you most.

A client who took to journaling immediately was Niles. Niles is not a true self-help kind of a guy, so his husband referred him to me because he felt Niles' eating was "getting out of control." Uncertain about most of the tools and techniques I was recommending, Niles was not sure I could help him until I suggested journaling. Niles loves to write. He wrote his vows for his wedding. He writes poetry in his spare time and like most Los Angelenos, he is trying his hand at a screenplay. A bit too young to have heard of Julia Cameron when she first hit the scene, Niles immediately ordered her book.

Every morning at 6:00 a.m., he would reach for his journal and write, stream of consciousness style, until three pages were filled. At first, he wrote about his day, his work, and his husband. But after a few weeks, his writing turned more towards his emotions, his upbringing, and his feeling about his weight. The daily writing sessions brought Niles more in touch with his emotions and himself. Soon he was journaling about the questions I gave out at the end of each TAME session. His insights about his relationship with food grew and he became more interested in the rest of the mindful eating program. A win for everyone.

GETTING EXTRA HELP

If your emotions overwhelm you, or if you have suffered a serious trauma or loss, please don't try to heal all by yourself. Ask for help. I encourage you to find a licensed mental health professional for assistance. The magazine *Psychology Today* has a website where you can find licensed psychologists in your area. If you have health insurance, you can go to the insurance company's website for referrals within your network. If you want a personal referral, ask your physician or trusted family friend. There is no shame in asking for assistance. Help is there for you if you seek it.

TAME Your Appetite is designed as a self-help program, but you don't have to do it that way. If you want help implementing the Steps, you have a few options. First you can find a few friends and create a study group. You can work through the Steps together offering support and encouragement.

Second, if you are working with a psychologist, you can bring her a copy of this book and work with it in your sessions.

Finally, you are welcome to contact me and participate in a *TAME Your Appetite* program. As I mentioned previously, the five steps you are learning here are based on my *TAME Your Appetite* programs, which are more extensive and experiential.

For more information, go to www.TAMEYourAppetite.com/Programs.

SOME MORE ABOUT CRAVINGS

As I mentioned previously, clients often complain to me about their cravings and I remind them that cravings can be handled with mindfulness. Here are some more tips on how to deal with them.

To manage cravings mindfully, try the following:

First, study your craving. Be curious about it. What does it feel like? Where in your body do you experience it? If it had a color, what color would it be? Can you give it a name? Is there a message inside your craving?

Is it telling you you are physically hungry? If you are physically hungry, decide what you are hungry for and eat. If what you are hungry for is what you are craving, enjoy a portion of it mindfully.

If you are not physically hungry, is it telling you that you are emotionally hungry? If you are emotionally hungry, identify your emotional need and address it as you learned about in this step.

If you are not physically or emotionally hungry and are experiencing a craving, ride it out. Give yourself twenty to thirty minutes to let it pass. Practice "Riding the Wave," using your craving as the focal point. The principle is the same as when you used this tool to help with your emotions. You can also do something else. Distract yourself. Sip a cup of tea.

Whatever you do in response to a craving, don't panic. Stay mindful and you will find your way through it.

STEP FOUR SUMMARY:

Meditation develops the skill of non-judgmental awareness, teaching us how to be with what is happening as it happens. This is extremely helpful in coping with emotions. As your meditation practice deepens, you may find that you not only deal with emotions like anger more easily, but you may also find that you are less emotional in general.

With meditation in your toolbox, you can learn to be with your emotions without acting on them. By allowing your feelings to come and go, they will eventually fade away without fanfare. Practice being with different emotions and, with compassion and gentleness, try not to react to them. Just be present. Rather than struggle against what you are feeling, be patient and kind with yourself. Make friends with your emotions and listen for how they are trying to help you. This will make it easier to stay with them instead of pushing them away. It may seem counterintuitive but staying with your feelings makes them go away faster than avoiding them does.

Use the meditation from this Step whenever you need help staying with your emotions. Practice identifying what else you can do to help yourself address what you really need. When we are mindless, we react to our emotions by eating. With mindfulness, you have an opportunity to be with the emotion, to accept it, and to learn from it.

> ### MINDFUL BITE:
>
> **Decide what you are really hungry for and then provide it for yourself. There is no better healing than that.**

Chapter Eight

Step Five – Expanding Mindfulness to the Rest of Your Life

There are only two ways to live your life. One is as though nothing is a miracle. The other is as though everything is a miracle.

Albert Einstein

Welcome to Step Five, the final step in this program. With this step, you will expand mindfulness into other areas of your life so you can experience more of the benefits a mindful approach to life can offer. By integrating mindfulness into your everyday activities such as cooking, washing dishes, and driving, you will have a chance to experience the effects of mindfulness on your health and overall well-being. In this step, we will pay special attention to how mindfulness helps with anxiety, sadness, pain, and insomnia. In addition, the Healing Self-Touch meditation will demonstrate how you can use meditation as a source of comfort. Finally, we will end with some tips on "getting good" at mindfulness.

USING MINDFULNESS IN EVERYDAY LIFE

A wonderful aspect of mindfulness is that it can be used anywhere at any time during any task. If we remember that mindfulness is simply paying attention in a non-judgmental way, we can see how it applies in all situations. Let's take cooking as an example.

MINDFUL COOKING

Mindful cooking is paying attention to each element of the process without distraction. Try it for yourself. Start by mindfully choosing a recipe to prepare. Sit down with your favorite cookbook and slowly leaf through it. Feel the pages under your fingertips. Linger over photos that may be included. Choose a recipe that calls out to you, one that is appetizing and enticing.

If you don't have any cookbooks or don't know where to start, here are three fabulous recipes to use. The first, *Aztec Guacamole*, is from my friend Karen Owoc, founder of www.athletesinaprons.com. The second, *Pan-Seared Salmon*, is adapted from a recipe I found inside a weekly circular from a favorite local market. It's amazing what you can discover when you pay attention! The third, *Grandma Charlotte's World-Famous Banana Bread*, is a cherished recipe from my mom. These simple recipes are great ones with which to begin your practice of mindful cooking or baking.

AZTEC GUACAMOLE ("BROCCAMOLE")

12 oz. broccoli florets
1 large avocado, pit removed, flesh scooped out
1 1/2 small limes, juiced
1/8 tsp. or less Hawaiian sea salt
1/2 c. cilantro, chopped (approximately 1/2 bunch)
3/4 c. Roma tomatoes, seeded and diced (approximately 1 1/2 tomatoes)
1/2 medium onion, chopped
1/2 jalapeno pepper, seeded and finely diced (reserve some seeds)
1 large clove garlic, crushed
A few drops of hot sauce (optional)

Steam the broccoli until tender and set aside. Chop the cilantro and Roma tomatoes and place in a medium bowl. Finely dice the onion and jalapeno peppers and add to the bowl. Add the minced garlic and, if desired, add a few drops of hot sauce and stir. Combine the steamed broccoli and avocado in a food processor and pulse very briefly. Add the lime juice and sea salt to the processor and pulse again to blend. If you want it authentic, keep it a bit chunky. Combine the ingredients from the food processor into the bowl and blend. Makes two cups.

MARKET FRESH PAN-SEARED SALMON

2 salmon fillets
2 tsp. olive oil
¼ tsp salt
fresh ground pepper

Wash the salmon fillets and pat dry. Brush each fillet with the oil and sprinkle with salt and pepper. Heat a non-stick sauté pan over medium heat. Place the fillets in the pan, flesh side down, and cook for two minutes. Turn the fillets over and cook for an additional two minutes. Position the cooked fillets onto a plate, loosely cover with aluminum foil for five minutes, and then serve. These fillets also taste great cold over a green salad.

GRANDMA CHARLOTTE'S WORLD-FAMOUS BANANA BREAD

1 1/3 cup flour
2 tsp. baking powder
¼ tsp. salt
1/3 cup canola oil
2/3 cup sugar
2 eggs
2–3 mashed (very ripe) bananas

Preheat oven to 350 degrees. Lightly coat a baking loaf pan with oil. Mix all the ingredients together in a bowl, using an electric mixer. If you don't have an electric mixer, use a wooden spoon and mix until all ingredients are blended. It may help to beat the eggs before adding them to the other ingredients if you are using a spoon. Pour the mixture into the loaf pan and bake for one hour. The banana bread will be golden brown on the outside and moist on the inside when it is done. To check if it is completely baked, stick a toothpick into the center of the loaf. If it comes out dry, the bread is done. If it is wet, bake a little longer until the toothpick comes out dry. Let cool and serve. This recipe will make 8 to 12 servings depending on how thick you cut the slices. A slice of this banana bread with a cup of tea or coffee is a fabulous meal or snack.

Once you have settled on a recipe, the next step is to mindfully prepare your shopping list if there are ingredients you need which you don't have. Make the shopping list only about this recipe. Exclude other items that you might need for your household. You can get them later. Your focus for the moment is on this recipe.

Now it's time to go shopping. (You can practice mindful driving on your way to the store by following the suggestions below.) Before you step into the store, take a deep breath and relax your body. Most of the time, we rush into the store, grab what we need, and leave. Today, you will savor your shopping experience. To do so, place your attention on the here and now. Take a full breath, exhale slowly, and begin your shopping excursion by taking a basket or cart. As you touch the basket or cart, feel it in your hands. Notice its weight, size, and color. Is it clean? Do you want to use this one or choose another? Next, look at your list. Take your time walking around the store and carefully choose your items. Place the items in your basket one by one, feeling their weight, and admiring their packaging or natural texture. When you have collected all your items, proceed to the checkout counter. Notice the other people in line. Take in the sights and sounds around you. Be present. Place your items one by one on the conveyor belt or counter and silently thank all those who helped get them to the store for your purchase. When it is your turn, acknowledge the cashier (and bagger, if there is one) and thank her for helping you today.

When you return home, thoughtfully place your ingredients on your kitchen counter or table and begin making the recipe. Tend to each instruction deliberately. Don't rush. Find the pleasure in the process.

While your recipe is cooking, baking, or cooling, set your table. Lay out beautiful dishes and flatware. Use crystal and china if you have it. Add flowers and candles if you like.

Serve the dish as you would expect the finest restaurant in the world to do. Savor each bite as if it were the first time you have ever tasted it. Bon Appetit.

WASHING DISHES MINDFULLY

When you are finished preparing the recipe above, it is time to wash the dishes. Washing dishes is an exceptionally good way to practice mindfulness. In Chapter Two, Being Mindful, I opened with a quote from Thich Nhat Hanh and told you about his experience as a Buddhist monk washing dishes. Here is the entire quote from his book, *The Miracle of Mindfulness: An Introduction to the Practice of Meditation.*

"While washing the dishes, one should only be washing the dishes, which means that while washing the dishes, one should be completely aware of the fact that one is washing the dishes. At first glance, that might seem a little silly: why put so much stress on a simple thing? But that's precisely the point. The fact that I am standing there and washing these bowls is a wondrous reality. I'm being completely myself, following my breath, conscious of my presence, and conscious of my thoughts and actions. There's no way I can be tossed around mindlessly like a bottle slapped here and there on the waves.

While washing dishes, you might be thinking about the tea you're going to drink afterwards, and so you try to get them out of the way as quickly as possible in order to sit and drink tea. But that means that you are incapable of living during the time you are washing the dishes. When you are washing the dishes, washing the dishes must be the most important thing in your life. Just as when you're drinking tea, drinking tea must be the most important thing in your life."

Take a lesson from the esteemed monk and when you wash your dishes, only wash the dishes.

MINDFULLY DRIVING

Unless you live in a major city like New York or Chicago, it is very likely you spend a lot of time driving in your car. Because we spend so much time in our cars, driving becomes a perfect opportunity to practice mindfulness. In fact, with millions of people getting killed or injured in car accidents every year, we could also argue that mindful driving is vital to our safety and well-being.

Let's begin with a look at what I mean by mindless driving. Think about your ordinary driving habits. Are you a mindless driver? Do you fail to be completely attentive to your driving? Or, in other words, is your mind somewhere else? It is not uncommon to drive for long stretches without being fully present. I am sure it has happened to you. For example, have you ever driven home from work and not remembered how you got there? Or passed an exit you always take? There is a phrase to describe this phenomenon. It is called Highway Hypnosis (also known as White Line Fever). Researchers explain it as a state of mind in which a person can drive long distances and not remember doing so. For our purposes, we will refer to this type of driving as mindless driving.

Other forms of mindless driving include driving while on the cell phone, listening to loud music, having a conversation with a passenger, shaving, putting on makeup, texting, drinking coffee, or eating lunch. (When I think I have seen it all, another driver passes by doing another totally mindless action!)

Your driving style can also reflect mindlessness. For instance, are you an aggressive driver, weaving in and out of traffic without regard for speed limits or other traffic laws? On the flip side, are you a nervous driver who hesitates when merging or entering intersections?

Mindful driving means paying attention to all facets of driving, and it starts before you turn on the ignition. Just like you get ready to begin a sitting meditation by finding the right position, setting your timer, eliminating distractions, and closing your eyes, when you get ready to drive, you need to prepare too.

It starts with your car. Is your car in good repair? Are the tires safe to drive on? Is there enough gasoline (or electric charge) to get you where you are going? Paying attention to these details is being mindful.

When you settle in behind the steering wheel, do as you do in sitting meditation and find a comfortable, relaxed position—one that keeps you alert and focused.

Next, move your bag or briefcase beyond your reach, turn off the radio, disconnect the Bluetooth, and leave your coffee mug in the kitchen sink. Mindful driving is undistracted driving. I can hear your objections already: "Without my coffee, radio, phone [you fill in the blank], my drive is boring, tedious, too long." Yes, I get it. But trust me, start with this amount of detail to your driving (like you did with the raisin exercise for mindful eating) and, as you become a more mindful driver, you will be able to listen to the radio and still be attentive. Mindful driving is a skill which you can develop with practice. Once you are mindfully in position, you are ready to drive. Take several deep breaths, start the engine, and go.

To keep your mind on your driving, use the steering wheel as you would your breath in a sitting meditation. Use the sensation of your hands on the steering wheel as focal point. If you are used to driving with only one hand on the wheel, see if you can break that habit and get used to a two-hand position. It is safer and gives you more control over the car. When your mind wanders away from the road (and it will, as you know by now), bring your attention to your hands and feel the steering wheel again. Notice if it is hard or soft. Are you gripping or relaxed? If your steering wheel offers temperature control, is it hot or cool? Feel the texture of the wheel in your hand. Sense the vibrations running through it from the engine. Keep coming back to the steering wheel whenever your mind wanders. Putting your attention on your hands brings you back to the present and able to put your mind back on the road.

John rushed into session breathless.

"What's wrong?" I asked.

"I almost had three accidents driving over here," he exclaimed.

"Sit down. Take a deep breath and tell me all about it," I instructed.

We spent the next forty-five minutes talking about his near misses. John takes surface streets to get to my office from his home, so fortunately he was not going fast as these incidents occurred.

The first one, he explained, happened when someone pulled out of an alley right in front of him. The other driver was "oblivious to me," John said. "Thank goodness, I was paying attention."

The next event happened just a minute later when someone drove right through a four-way stop. John had gotten to the signs first and stopped.

He explained: "The other driver was to my left and came barreling past me at least fifty miles an hour in a residential area! Can you believe it? If I hadn't stopped, I'd be a goner now," John said as he shook his head.

"Thank goodness I was paying attention," he repeated.

The last instance was the most frightening for him.

"She came out of nowhere," he said, describing a pedestrian who seemed to suddenly appear in front of his moving car.

"She was wearing a headset," he continued, "and came out into the street between two parked cars. I slammed on my breaks as I blasted my horn. That got her attention," he said as he finally relaxed into his chair. "Thank goodness I was paying attention," he uttered again.

"It is a good thing you were paying attention," I replied. "In fact, it was good thing you were paying attention each time, or the circumstances could have been much worse."

I paused to give John some time to think about what I had just said.

He grinned and said, "I guess I was the mindful one!"

"Indeed, you were," I said, smiling back.

How many times have you had "near-misses"? Or more correctly, "near-hits"? How many times were you the one paying attention and how many times were you the one causing the potential problem? One moment of mindlessness while driving, or even while being the pedestrian, can have dire consequences. Practice mindfulness while driving (and walking) for a happier, healthier, and potentially longer life.

EVERYDAY MINDFULNESS—ONE TASK AT A TIME

Mindfulness can be practiced at any time, in any situation. All it takes is a willingness to stay present, to intentionally pay attention and to ascribe no judgement to what is occurring in the moment. Mindfulness is being with what is. You can practice everyday mindfulness by choosing to be present, choosing to keep your attention in the here and now, and choosing to get the most from each activity and interaction, whether you are eating, driving, walking, or washing the dishes. By simply slowing down, you will become more mindful. It can be as easy as that.

In the next chapter, I will show you how you can deepen your mindfulness practice and strengthen your mindful eating habits with a daylong retreat. But, before we go there, let's review some of the health benefits that a mindfulness meditation practice can produce.

THE HEALTH BENEFITS OF MINDFULNESS MEDITATION

A quick Google search of the term "health benefits of mindfulness meditation" yielded over a half million hits. If you are a science geek, you are welcome to read them all. If you are not, let me summarize them for you.

Among the physical health benefits that research has demonstrated occur because of meditation are:

- Increased immune function;
- Increased cortical thickness (that means more gray matter in your brain);
- Improved memory, focus and attention;
- Improved sleep; and
- Decreased pain and inflammation.

As for the psychological health benefits of meditation, research shows us that it:

- Decreases anxiety, stress and depression;
- Increases positive effect (that means you're in a better mood);
- Increases emotional intelligence (that means you have better people skills);
- Increases compassion for self and others; and
- Increases emotional regulation (meaning you have more control over your emotions).

Let's takes a closer look at some of the conditions that may affect your weight and how a regular meditation practice can positively impact them. We will start with a common woe, anxiety.

USING MINDFULNESS TO HEAL THE FEAR-FILLED MIND

Anxiety is fear of the future. You feel anxious when you anticipate something bad happening. The something bad could be real, requiring your immediate attention, or it could be imaginary ("noise" as some psychologists like to call it). Learning to differentiate between real and imagined anxiety is an important skill and mindfulness can help you do that. (I also address how to learn the difference between real and imagined anxiety in my book, *The Best Diet Begins in Your Mind*. You might want to take a look there for extra assistance.)

The truth is, we are all anxious from time to time and that is not a bad thing. Anxiety can alert us to danger. Problems arise when are persistently anxious for no good reason and we use food to avoid or distract ourselves from it. Acquiring a better way to manage your anxiety is where mindfulness comes in.

Anxiety is felt in both the body and the mind. Some of the physical symptoms of anxiety include heart palpitations, sweating, upset stomach, headaches, dizziness, and high blood pressure. Our mind can be affected by anxiety in the form of frightening thoughts, feelings of dread, the desire to flee, and the inability to do anything (we freeze). Mindfulness helps us recognize both types of symptoms.

With a mindfulness meditation practice, you come to understand how your body and your mind react to anxiety. Through your practice, you can detect the mechanism by which your mind takes what is happening in the present and leads you to a dark and horrible future. You watch as your mind leaves the current moment and carries you off into fantasies. By observing your thoughts and not attaching to them, you can separate from them. You develop the ability to stay with the anxious thoughts and feelings without acting on them. By staying with the anxiety, you transform it. In essence, you learn to be with your fears without being afraid of them. They become merely thoughts that float through your mind and back out again, like any other thought you might think. The more you practice being with your anxious thoughts, the less you will need to eat to quell your anxiety, and your food intake will naturally decrease.

Here's a short meditation to show you how to detach from your anxious thoughts:

Begin by sitting with a relaxed but straight posture. Loosen any tight clothing. Rest your hands in your lap and gently close your eyes. Focus your mind on the feeling of your breathing. Take two deep breaths, letting the air flow all the way into your stomach and then flow gently back out again. Let your breathing find its own natural, comfortable rhythm.

As you continue, you may notice your mind getting caught up in thoughts about the future. This is fine. This is what the mind does. When you notice your mind fantasizing about the future, simply observe it. Without any judgement of yourself for having these thoughts or any judgement about the thoughts themselves, merely witness your mind as it thinks them. Acknowledge your mind for doing what minds do and then return your attention to your breath. Ride the flow of the breath, feeling it move in and out with a gentle, natural rhythm.

Whenever your mind wanders to the future, note that this is happening and return to your breath. Each time you do so, you are detaching from the thoughts and releasing the anxiety they carry.

Continue to be with your breath and when you are ready, gently bring your attention back into the room and open your eyes.

THE THREE-MINUTE BREATHING SPACE MEDITATION

There is another meditation that you may find useful when dealing with stress and anxiety. It comes from a mindfulness-based psychotherapy treatment called Mindfulness-Based Cognitive Therapy (MBCT). Its purpose is to move you from distressing thoughts that are causing your stress and anxiety back to the present moment. It only takes three minutes and can be done anywhere, at any time. Here's how you do it:

Like any other meditation, you begin by getting centered and, if possible, close your eyes. Turn your attention inward and ask yourself "what is going on inside of me right now?" What are you thinking? Feeling? Any bodily sensations? Then, you move your attention to your breath only. Spend a minute or so with your breath the way you do in other breathing meditations. Focus on the movement and sensation of the breath in the body and when your mind wanders, redirect it back to the breath. Next, shift your attention to your whole body, as if your whole body were breathing. Get a sense of your entire body. If a particular part of your body grabs your attention, breathe into it and then return to the whole body. To end the meditation, open your awareness to all that is around you, to your entire life, and when you are ready open your eyes.

Practice this Three-Minute Breathing Space meditation throughout the day whenever you start to feel overwhelmed or frightened. The effects are cumulative.

If you are interested in a full course using mindfulness to manage stress and anxiety, look for a Mindfulness-Based Stress Reduction (MBSR) program. MBSR, created by Jon Kabat-Zinn, is the first and most widely studied mindfulness treatment protocol. MBSR set the stage for other mindfulness-based syllabi, including MB-EAT, upon which this program is based. MBSR is typically offered as an eight-week program with a forty-five-minute daily meditation component and a half-day retreat.

There is another meditation I would like to introduce that can be used when you are feeling out of sorts. It is called the Healing Self-Touch Meditation.

HEALING SELF-TOUCH MEDITATION

Did you know that babies die if they are not touched? This phenomenon is known as "Failure to Thrive Syndrome." We hear it occurring in orphanages in under-developed countries where they do not have the resources to provide adequate care to newborns. As adults, we need to be touched too. We may not die if we are not touched, but touch can be very soothing—even our own touch. I will now guide you through the meditation called "Healing

Self-Touch." This meditation can be effective when you are feeling anxious because it provides comfort and calming.

> Take a moment to position yourself comfortably. Take several deep breaths and, when you are ready, close your eyes.
>
> Now bring your awareness to your hands and notice what they are touching. Maybe they are in your lap and you can feel the weight of your hands on your legs. Or maybe your hands are clasped. Feel your fingers intertwined. If they are resting on the arms of the chair, feel its texture. Notice whatever sensations are present. Take a few deep breaths, resting your attention on your hands.
>
> Wherever your hands are, gently turn them so that your palms are facing up. If you want to move them into another position, feel free to do so mindfully. If your mind becomes cluttered by chatter, simply let that chatter go and come back to your hands.
>
> Now, imagine your hands are filling up with kindness. Imagine they are full of caring, warmth, and tenderness.
>
> Now, gently, lift one hand up and lightly place it on the opposite arm. Notice what this feels like, the sensation of touching. Notice your response. Now do the same with the other arm as if you are giving yourself a soft hug. Keep your hands cradled on your arms and notice what comes up. How does it feel to touch yourself so delicately?
>
> Now, shift your awareness from the top of your arms to deeper center, to the bones which give your arms strength and to the muscles which allow them to move and hold things.
>
> As you do this, what is going through your mind? Notice without judgement the thoughts that arise. If unwanted thoughts or feelings show up, notice them, and let them flow away as you redirect your focus to your arms.
>
> If you like, you may gently rub your arms, caressing them with a loving touch. Stay aware of both the surface and the core of your body.
>
> When you are ready, move both hands, still filled with kindness, to your thighs, gently placing them wherever is comfortable and relaxing. Allow any feelings of tenderness to surface.
>
> Now gently caress your thighs and further down your legs if you wish. Notice your response.
>
> Slowly move your hands onto your stomach, resting with the movement of your stomach as you breathe. Continue to feel the kindness cupped in your hands. Notice your response.

Finally, place one hand over your heart. If you can, notice your heart-beat. Feel your heart's caring nature in your hand.

As we come to the close of this meditation, your hands can remain where they are or, if you prefer, you can move them to wherever your body might need a loving touch. Mindfully move your hands to that spot and rest them there with a sense of warmth and appreciation.

And now bring your awareness back to your breath. Slowly bring your attention back into the room and, when you're ready, open your eyes.

THE MINDFUL WAY OUT OF SADNESS

Whether we miss a friend who has moved away or are just having a bad day, sadness affects all of us at one time or another. Sadness can last for moments, hours, or even days, depending on the cause. When we are sad, we tend to shut down. We do what we can to avoid the feelings that accompany our mood. We turn away from what is bothering us and often turn towards food for relief. Besides bad feelings, another characteristic of sadness and depression is negative thinking. Our minds become filled with negative thoughts which we believe to be true. We ruminate over the notion that things will never get better. Such beliefs perpetuate our down mood.

Depression is a serious form of sadness. It is one that affects us more profoundly than sadness and can last for years if untreated. True depression is a psychological and medical matter that requires intervention. It goes without saying, if you are experiencing depression, please get the right kind of professional help. Mindfulness-Based Cognitive Therapy (MBCT), mentioned earlier, is an excellent option, as is traditional psychotherapy and, if appropriate, medication. You can use mindfulness meditation in conjunction with these treatments to increase their benefits.

Mindfulness has been shown to help alleviate both sadness and depression in three ways. First, mindfulness helps us recover from sadness by turning our attention towards our feelings. Like with anxiety, we learn to be with the feelings rather than escape them. By getting centered and noticing what is happening in the body and mind, we move towards our pain rather than away from it. Mindfulness practices connect us to our feelings and help us feel compassion towards ourselves.

Second, mindfulness teaches us to observe our negative thoughts without getting attached to them. We gain a different perspective on the thoughts that fuel the depressive state and see how they can pass by us without taking up residency in our minds. By redirecting our attention to the present, we can release these thoughts.

Third, when we are feeling sad or depressed, we often feel as if we have entered a dark place. Our mood envelops us, and we might feel as if there is no way out, as if we may not survive. This is especially true for both clinical depression and protracted grief. To get relief, it becomes important to be able to be in the dark places and not feel as if we will perish. Mindfulness allows us to enter these states, observe them and then let them go.

What follows is a brief meditation to show you how to be with your sadness and depression:

Begin by sitting with a relaxed but straight posture. Loosen any tight clothing. Rest your hands in your lap and gently close your eyes. Focus your mind on the feeling of your breathing. Take two deep breaths, letting the air flow all the way into your stomach and then flow gently back out again. Let your breathing find its own natural, comfortable rhythm. As you continue, notice the emotional discomfort within your body. Draw your attention to that discomfort and breathe deeply. Be with the discomfort as you breathe in and out, in and out. Do this without judgement. Allow yourself to feel compassion for yourself and your body.

If your mind gets caught up in negative thoughts or feeling, it's okay. This is the nature of the mind. When you notice the negative thoughts, simply observe them. Without any judgement of yourself for having these thoughts or any judgement about the thoughts themselves, watch your mind as it thinks these thoughts. Acknowledge your mind for doing what minds do and then return your attention to your breath. Ride the flow of breath, feeling it move in and out with a gentle, natural rhythm.

Whenever bodily sensations arise or your mind strays into the negative, note that this is happening and return to your breath. Each time you do so, you are detaching from the thoughts and releasing emotional pain.

Continue to be with your breath for as long as you like and when you are ready, gently bring your attention back into the room and open your eyes.

Use this meditation anytime you are feeling blue. It will restore your mood and help you avoid eating in response to your sadness.

ATTENDING TO PAIN THE MINDFUL WAY

It may not surprise you to learn that the research investigating physical pain is looking at the mind-body connection for answers. Chronic pain is being studied as a stress-related medical condition. If we use chronic back pain as an example, researchers are discovering that this type of pain has less to do with actual damage to the spinal cord and more to do with muscle tension. Furthermore, the negative thoughts we have about pain when we experience it exacerbates the problem, causing more stress, and leading to more pain. A vicious cycle ensues. Luckily, mindfulness offers a solution.

You may be familiar with the famous adage "pain is inevitable, but suffering is optional." The truth is you cannot avoid pain. We all get hurt at one time or another. You cannot control that. Suffering, on the other hand, is brought about by evaluating and resisting the pain. You may not be able to prevent pain, but you can control your reaction to it. This is where mindfulness comes in.

With mindfulness, we learn to separate physical pain from emotional suffering. The negative commentary, the prayers for relief, the anger, and the fear all contribute to the continuation of the discomfort. Instead of shunning the pain or complaining about it, we mindfully choose to turn our attention to it. By watching the mind, we can see how our thoughts contribute to our pain. By turning our attention toward the pain, we can notice that pain is not stagnant. We observe how it changes, ebbs and flows, and comes and goes.

Research conducted on the effects of meditation on pain concluded that experienced meditators experience pain differently than new or non-meditators. Specifically, researchers found that experienced meditators felt pain less acutely because they evaluated and resisted their pain less.

Let me guide you through a brief meditation that can help you with chronic pain.

MINDFUL PAIN MEDITATION

Start by getting into a comfortable position. If sitting hurts too much, lie down. Try to get as comfortable as possible, given any limitations you may be dealing with. Take a few breaths and connect with your body.

We will begin by finding a part of your body that is not in pain. Bring your attention to it. If you cannot find a part that has no pain, find one that feels pleasant or even neutral. Let your attention rest at that part for a few moments.

Now bring your attention to the area of your body where you feel pain. What do you detect? Is the pain severe? It is sharp or dull? Burning? Stabbing? Piercing? Shooting? Cramping? Is it in one place? Is it moving? How deep does it go or is it on the surface? Be curious about your pain and the changing sensations.

Stay with your pain for as long as you can. Then move your attention back to the neutral body part. Rest there for a minute or two and when you are ready return to the painful part.

How do you feel about the pain? Are you angry? Are you afraid of it? Are you resentful? Annoyed? Embarrassed? Ashamed? Are there any physical sensations? Notice what is there, breathe, and let it be.

Return your attention to the neutral area, and once again remain there for a minute or so.

Now, for the last time, return to the painful spot. What do you notice now? Offer yourself some kindness and compassion. Does anything change?

When you are ready, bring your attention to your whole body, back to the room in which you are sitting or lying and open your eyes.

If you want to read more about using mindfulness to manage pain, check out *Fully Present: The Science, Art, and Practice of Mindfulness* by Susan Smalley and Diana Winston, and *You Are Not Your Pain* by Vidyamala Burch and Danny Penman.

MINDFUL ZZZZ'S

If you have a hard time sleepihg, I have some good news for you. Mindfulness practices have proven to be an effective treatment for insomnia. So, whether your insomnia shows up as trouble falling asleep, waking up in the middle of the night with difficulty going back to sleep, or waking up too early and struggling to sleep until your desired wake-up time, mindfulness meditation can help.

It is important to our physical and psychological health that we sleep well each night. We are a nation, probably a world, of sleep-deprived people. Most of us think this is just how it is and fuel up on excess caffeine and food to get through the day. Powering through the day is not the answer. Insomnia is a big problem. Insomnia is more than just an inconvenience because lack of sleep can cause impairment in our thinking, increased susceptibility to illness, high blood pressure, dependence on sleep medication, injuries, car accidents, and absences from work and life.

Typical treatments for insomnia are prescription and over-the-counter medications and herbal and other alternative supplements. I would like to offer another option—Mindfulness-Based Therapy for Insomnia (MBTI).

Based on the work of Jason C. Ong, Ph.D., Associate Professor in the Department of Neurology at Northwestern University Feinberg School of Medicine, and author of *Mindfulness-Based Therapy for Insomnia*, MBTI restores good sleep by shifting the person's relationship to the thoughts and behaviors she has about sleep. Rather than changing thoughts about sleep, MBTI instructs the person to observe her thoughts about sleep and to allow the brain to restore sleep itself without force or striving.

Using meditation as a foundation, MBTI results in a greater awareness of the thoughts which contribute to sleeplessness, such as "I need eight hours every night or I can't function the next day," "I'll never get my work done if I don't sleep," "I can't take this sleeplessness anymore," "All I want to do is sleep!" and "I'm so depressed and angry that I am not sleeping." By cultivating awareness of these thoughts, you increase your understanding of the mental and physical states that arise when you are experiencing insomnia and learn how to shift your responses to them.

Here are some tips on mindful sleep habits derived from my audio/visual version of MBTI called Sound Mind, Sound Sleep, which is available through the store at TAMEYourAppetite.com/shop. Please think of these tips as your initial steps towards developing awareness of your sleep habits.

1   Regularize the time that you go to bed and get out of bed so that the amount of time you spend in bed is consistent.

2   Avoid putting effort into trying to sleep. Increased effort is likely to make you more anxious and frustrated rather than sleepy. Only go to sleep when you are sleepy.

3   Avoid caffeine, alcohol, and nicotine starting from the late afternoon or early evening.

4   Get regular, moderate exercise daily, but avoid exercising too close to bedtime. Do not attempt to use exercise to "tire yourself out."

5   Avoid late meals and middle of the night eating. If you are physically hungry, a light snack at bedtime is not likely to negatively impact your sleep.

6   Make your sleep environment comfortable. For example, use an eye mask to reduce light exposure and a fan or white noise generator to reduce sound.

7   You can also end each day with a Body Scan Meditation to relax your body and mind.

BODY SCAN MEDITATION

This meditation is typically done lying down, but feel free to choose any position that suits your body. I thank Dr. Kristeller for some of the language in this meditation.

Become comfortable and relaxed. Find a position so that you will not become drowsy but that is comfortable, not straining.

Allow your body to become still. Focus your mind on the feeling of your breathing. Begin by taking in two or three deeper breaths. Notice an increased sense of calm and relaxation as you breathe in the clean, fresh air and breathe out any tension or stress, letting your breathing find its own natural, comfortable rhythm and depth.

Now bring your awareness to your whole body and notice any physical sensations that arise, such as itchiness, tension, tightness, or pain. If physical sensations are present, try bringing awareness to the sensation rather than trying to make it go away. Notice if there are any parts of your body which feel neutral to you.

Now, bring your awareness to your left foot. Bring full awareness to this part of your body. Notice all of the sensations that are present without judgement. Take a mindful breath and relax.

Now, bring your awareness to your left leg. Bring full awareness to this part of your body. Notice all of the sensations that are present without judgement. Take a mindful breath and relax.

Now allow your awareness to shift from the left leg to the right foot. Again, bring full awareness to this part of the body, noting all the sensations that are present, without judgement.

As you continue, you will notice that the mind will become caught up with thoughts and feelings. It may become attached to sensations or sounds. This is to be expected. This is the nature of the mind. When you notice this—without self-judgment—simply observe the process of the mind, then return your attention to your body.

Now allow your awareness to move to the right leg. Again, bring full awareness to this part of the body, noting all of the sensations that are present without judgement. Relax.

If your mind wanders, simply observe the process of the mind, then return your attention back to your right leg.

Now bring your awareness from your right leg to your back. Bring full awareness to this part of your body. Notice all of the sensations that are present without judgement. Take a mindful breath and relax.

Now allow your awareness to withdraw from your back and move it to your torso. Again, bring full awareness to this part of the body, noting all of the sensations that are present without judgement. Take a deep breath and relax.

Now, shift your awareness from your torso to your shoulders. Bring full awareness to this part of your body. Notice all of the sensations that are present without judgement. Take a mindful breath and relax.

If your mind becomes attached to thoughts or sounds, simply observe the process of the mind, then return your attention to your shoulders.

Now allow your awareness to move from your shoulders to your head. Again, bring full awareness to this part of the body, noting all of the sensations that are present, without judgement. Take a mindful breath and relax.

Now, bring your awareness to your entire body. Notice all of the sensations that are present, without judgement. Take a mindful breath and relax.

Now shift your awareness to the connection among all your different body parts. Again, bring full awareness to these connections, without judgement. Relax into these connections.

As we bring this meditation to an end, thank your body for any communication or new awareness that may have occurred during this meditation.

Slowly bring your awareness back to your breath and into the space of this room. Gently move your body and, when you are ready, open your eyes.

This is a lovely meditation to do any time you want to feel connected to your body.

GETTING GOOD AT MINDFULNESS

The meditations and mindful eating practices I have been sharing with you are what are known as "formal practices." There are also "informal practices." Informal practices are those moments throughout the day when we choose to be more aware of our surroundings and circumstances than we might otherwise be. For example, when brushing our teeth.

If you are like me, you dutifully brush your teeth every morning and every evening. It is a task we do automatically, with very little forethought other than to grab the toothbrush and slap some toothpaste on it. While I am brushing my teeth, my mind is usually on other things. Events of the day. Tasks for tomorrow. Last minute chores before bed. But tooth brushing time could be a time for an informal mindfulness exercise. If you choose to focus your attention on the brushing and only the brushing, you are being mindful. Instead of reviewing your "To Do List," you focus on the experience of brushing your teeth. You feel the brush in your hand and against your teeth and gums. You taste the mint flavor of the toothpaste and the fresh clean water you use to rinse. You notice the foam as it fills your mouth and watch as it slips down the drain when you are done. If you floss, you can give the procedure your full attention as you swipe the thread around each tooth. For the two minutes dentists tell us to brush our teeth, we could be practicing two minutes of mindfulness.

You can pay the same kind of attention when you make your morning coffee or load up your backpack. These may not seem significant, but informal mindfulness practices repeated throughout the day make a difference. A strong informal practice strengthens your formal practice without your even trying.

More examples of when you can practice informal mindfulness include unloading the dishwasher, doing the laundry, walking the dog, and cutting vegetables.

There are also other times during the day that I sometimes use to practice mindfulness informally. They are when I am at a traffic light, when I am on hold on the phone, and when I am in line at the grocery store. In the past, these events would have frustrated me. Thoughts like "I don't have time for this" would fill my mind, making me agitated if I really had to be somewhere or needed to get something important done. Now, I have reframed these events as opportunities to practice being with whatever is. No one notices when I am doing this, and it has a gentle calming effect. Here's what I do:

When I am at a light, I look at the cars, people, buildings, and nature around me. I see new stores and restaurants that I might never have noticed if I wasn't being mindful at that moment. If a song is playing on the radio, I listen more closely. If a catering truck is nearby, I enjoy its aroma.

When I am on hold and there is music playing, I focus my attention on the melody, letting my breath rise and fall in sync. If there is no music, I sit, close my eyes and focus on my breathing until someone answers. When I do that, I am usually more patient with whatever comes next.

At the grocery store, I focus on the items in my cart. I count them as I lay them on the conveyor belt, touching each one and noting its color, weight, and size. Silly I know, but very centering. Much better for me than tapping my foot in aggravation.

Airports are another great place to practice informal mindfulness because there is so much going on, you can be present in so many ways. As you can probably tell, I am a people person. I love watching other travelers when I am waiting for a plane. I wonder where they are going and what they will do when they get there. I notice the clothes they are wearing and the food they are eating. I hear accents and foreign languages. In other words, I am fully present in my environment, taking in all the sights and sounds. If, however, you feel overstimulated at an airport because of all the people, noise, smells, and colors surrounding you, go within. Practice drawing your attention away from what is going on around you and focus on your breath as it moves in and out of your body.

Whether you engage in formal or informal mindfulness practices, getting good at being mindful requires only two things: an intention to be mindful and practice. You can do this. Melanie finally did.

My client Melanie resisted meditation from the first day I met her. A high-level executive with an MBA from a prestigious graduate school, Melanie told me her "mind wasn't wired for meditation." She said her mind works so fast "by necessity." She credited her success to her "remarkable mind." I agree that Melanie's mind is remarkable.

I believe that we all have remarkable minds and that, through mindfulness meditation, our minds can become even more remarkable. Melanie wasn't having any of it. She was interested in mindful eating and how it could help her lose the thirty pounds she's been carrying since her second child was born but wasn't going to "waste time on a cushion." Fair enough.

Since Melanie wasn't interested in a formal mindfulness practice, I introduced her to the idea of an informal one. I encouraged Melanie to practice everyday mindfulness. We began by making a list of several activities she did every day. Her list was making coffee, showering, styling her hair, and driving to work. I asked her which of these activities she would like to begin a mindfulness practice around. She chose making coffee.

Borrowing from Thich Nhat Hanh, I instructed Melanie to "only make coffee when she was making coffee." From pulling a filter out of the package, to measuring the coffee and the water, Melanie's attention was to be only on her coffee. No emails. No phone calls. No conversations with her husband or kids. While the coffee was brewing, Melanie was to continue to focus on the coffee experience. She was to smell the aroma as the coffee brewed. She was to feel the cool ceramic of her mug in her hand, admire the whiteness of the cream she poured in, and acknowledge the farmers, harvesters, roasters, and sellers who got her coffee to her.

The first time she did this, she scoffed. She said she felt silly, and her family rolled their collective eyes at her.

"No worries," I told her, "Keep doing it."

She did, every morning for a week. By the fourth day, her daughter was joining her in her ritual. Not a coffee drinker because she is only eleven, she mindfully prepared a glass of chocolate milk. When both beverages were ready, mother and daughter sat silently at their kitchen table, mindfully sipping their drinks.

When Melanie returned for her next mindful eating session, she was ready to add another mindful activity to her day. Each week, for the next month, Melanie added another everyday mindful activity. At the end of the month, Melanie reported that she was "naturally being more mindful" throughout her day. She noticed she had more patience for her subordinates and her family. She described feeling calmer and more focused. When one of her mindful eating cohorts asked if she was ready to try meditating, she happily said yes.

STEP FIVE SUMMARY:

Mindfulness is a powerful tool for increasing wellness and overall happiness and for decreasing pain and suffering. By applying it to specific situations, you can shift your experience and create something beneficial. If you suffer with anxiety, sadness, pain, or insomnia, practice the formal meditations provided on a daily basis to get relief. If you are not bothered by these issues, then adopt an informal approach by practicing mindfulness with everyday occurrences, such as washing dishes, cooking, and driving. In either case, I recommend you incorporate the Body Scan, Healing Self-Touch, and Three-Minute Breathing meditations into your routine. These three practices alone can make a difference in the quality of your life.

The most important thing about mindfulness is that you do it. You can spend a lifetime studying about it, reading about it, talking about it, and thinking about it, but until you do it, it won't do you (or your eating) any good. It can be hard to start being mindful. We are so conditioned to live our lives mindlessly that, in the beginning, it takes concerted effort. And once begun, it can sometimes feel difficult to continue, but when you do, the benefits are endless.

MINDFUL BITE:

A mindful life is a well-lived life.

Chapter Nine
A Day of Mindfulness

Mindfulness practice means that we commit fully in each moment to be present.

Jon Kabat-Zinn

As part of my training to become an MB-EAT Instructor, I attended several meditation retreats. A retreat is like a conference, except it is mostly silent. Retreats can take place over a day, a weekend, or several weeks. The purpose of these retreats is to be in the company of like-minded people and have the opportunity to do extensive meditation practices. The activities vary from retreat to retreat, but most incorporate sitting, walking, and eating meditations.

My very first meditation retreat was part of a series of classes I took through the Mindfulness Awareness Research Center (MARC) at UCLA. It was a half-day event and we met in the same location we had been using for our meditation classes. The instructions going into the retreat were quite simple. When we arrived, we were to take a seat on a chair or cushion and not talk. I must admit, I was a bit nervous heading over to the center. I had never been to a silent retreat before and didn't know what to expect. Turns out my fellow classmates were a bit anxious too, although I didn't know that until the end of the retreat when we were allowed to talk again.

When I arrived, I took the same seat I usually sat in and waited. As the others showed up, they did the same. Our teacher was already sitting in silence as the group assembled. Over the next four hours, she guided us through the various sitting meditations she taught us during the course. These included breathing, self-compassion, and healing touch meditations. Interspersed among the sitting meditations were opportunities to walk and gently move. I welcomed those respites because my body was achy from all the sitting.

At the conclusion of the retreat, we spent some time sharing what the event was like for each of us. Without exception, each person commented on their surprise over how pleasant it was and how much deeper their meditation practices felt. I took several more classes with this instructor and others and each included a silent retreat. By the time I got to my fourth one, I knew what to expect. That is, until I enrolled in a three-day silent retreat. That one was more intense.

The three-day retreat took place at a beautiful retreat center in central California, near Sacramento. The focus of this retreat was mindful eating so, on the way to the retreat center, I had to go shopping for food supplies. I was instructed to bring food for myself for two breakfasts, two lunches and one dinner, and to bring what I needed to prepare a dish to be shared with the other retreat-goers as part of a community meal. This retreat was very structured and included sitting meditations, yoga sessions, walking meditations, and information sessions. It was only during the information sessions that we were permitted to talk. The rest of the weekend took place in silence.

The setting was magnificent. Nestled in a lush valley, there were walking trails and other paths. The vista was also beautiful. During downtime, I sat with my journal looking out toward the valley and watched wild turkeys and other small critters do their nature thing. As a city girl, I found this quite appealing. At first, I felt all the silence to be disconcerting, but after the first day, I settled into the quiet and enjoyed the chance to go inward and learn about myself and how my mind works. Even though we rarely spoke to each other, I found myself bonding with the other seven women in attendance. Our shared experience drew us together.

My favorite part was the communal meal. It occurred on our last day. In preparing for the meal, the eight of us worked in silence in the community kitchen. We shared pots and pans, bowls, and spoons, without saying a word. We displayed our offerings on a buffet-style table and put little notes next to each dish describing its contents. When all the food was displayed, we assembled together, served ourselves what we wanted, and sat at a long table. At first, we ate in silence. Then, about halfway through the meal, we were invited to talk. As you can imagine, the chatter was lively. We discussed the food choices and their ingredients. We discussed who made what and why. We promised to share recipes when we got home.

After the meal, we talked about the difference we noticed between eating in silence and eating while talking. The general consensus was that when we started talking, we were less aware of the food, ate more, and tasted less. Since you are now a student of mindful eating, that revelation should not come as a surprise to you.

I have since done several day-long retreats. Some were part of training classes I took. Others were organized by local meditation centers. If a retreat interests you, join the email lists for meditation centers near you to learn when they are hosting such retreats. If you have the chance to go on one, I highly recommend it. Spending time with people who are also interested in mindfulness is wonderful. Being in silence is healing, once you get used to it. Also, having different teachers is a good idea. Their unique styles will expose you to different ways of being mindful and some may be better fits for you than others.

HOW TO CHOOSE A RETREAT

If my description of my retreat experience intrigued you, you might want to find a retreat to attend. Here's what I think you need to know to pick the right retreat for you.

First, you want to think about what kind of setting you would prefer. Do you want to be in the city or the mountains? Do you want to talk or be silent? Do you want it to be vegan, vegetarian, or some other menu? Do you want to sit in a chair or on cushions? Do you prefer to lie down? Finally, how long do you want the retreat to be? Half a day? Full day? Weekend? Weeklong?

You also want to assess the level of experience that the retreat leaders are expecting from participants. Think about where you are in your meditation journey and whether it matches what the retreat offers.

Next, who are the teachers? Is there only one? Or will you able to practice with many? If you are already taking meditation classes and this retreat is offered by your teacher, you already know her. But if you are considering a retreat offered by someone you do not know, do some homework. Find out who the teachers are and what their values and philosophies are. If a teacher is accessible, you might want to talk to him for more information.

I also suggest you set an intention for yourself with regard to the retreat. Ask yourself why you are going. What are you hoping to learn, feel, or do? At the same time, it is important to manage your expectations. It is unlikely you will become totally enlightened after one weekend retreat! But maybe you will improve your posture so you can sit longer in your practice. Or maybe you will meet a friend who can grow as meditator along with you.

There is one caveat I need to advise you of before enrolling in a retreat. If you are currently under significant emotional distress, or if your depression or anxiety is through the roof, discuss the retreat with your mental health practitioner. Make sure that this is the right time for you to take on such an endeavor.

YOUR OWN DAY OF MINDFULNESS

If getting to a retreat is not an option for you, you can create your own. To set up your own retreat, you simply dedicate a period of time to practice mindfulness in the comfort of your own home. Choose a day when you can be alone for a few hours. Send the kids, spouse, roommates, dogs, cats, and in-laws away for the duration. This is your time for peace and quiet. Set aside two to four hours when you do nothing but practice mindfulness by alternating among sitting, walking, and eating meditations.

To prepare for your retreat, here's what you do:

1   Pick a day and time that works for you.

2   Tell those close to you that you will be spending that time alone and ask them for privacy.

3   Prepare a schedule for your retreat. I will share a sample schedule.

4   Designate a room or area which will be the central point for your retreat. It could be a bedroom, den, patio, or garden. Choose whatever suits you best.

5   Make a list of any items you may need, including ingredients for whatever food you will be eating.

6   Go shopping for any items you are missing.

7   If you are going to do a walking meditation outside, choose your location. Make sure it is safe and convenient.

8   Get a good night's sleep the night before. If you can't because you are nervous, no worries, insomnia happens. You'll still be fine.

On the day of your retreat:

1   Kiss your loved ones good-bye and take a moment to be with the silence.

2   Assemble your meditation materials, including any guided meditation audios if you are using them, a timer, your cushion or chair, a blanket if you get cold, and anything else that you use as part of your practice.

3   Place your meditation materials in your designated space. Position candles and incense around if you like those things.

4   Organize the ingredients for the meals or snacks you will be eating during your retreat.

5   Have water or tea available.

6   If you want to do some yoga or light stretching as part of a moving meditation, place your mat or towel nearby.

7   When you are ready, begin your retreat.

Here is a suggested schedule which you can follow:

1   Begin your retreat with a sitting meditation. Try to make the length of this meditation thirty minutes, but if thirty minutes seems too long (or too short) adjust the time to suit your needs. Use a simple breathing meditation for this practice. Make your breath the focus. When your mind wanders, simply return it to your breath. You can do a silent or guided meditation, whichever you prefer.

2 After finishing your sitting meditation, mindfully prepare your first meal of the retreat. Depending upon when you start, this may be break-fast, lunch, or dinner. Be present for each step of the meal, from retriev-ing the food from the refrigerator, to slicing and dicing, to plating and serving. Think of your actions as sacred and treasured. Take your time. Eat slowly. Savor each bite and acknowledge all who helped you have this meal.

3 After eating, mindfully put your dishes and utensils away. If they re-quire washing, wash them as Thich Nhat Hanh would.

4 For the next part of your retreat do a walking meditation. For fifteen minutes (or whatever amount of time feels right for you), take a walk. When you walk, only walk. No cellphone. No iPod. Only walk. Pay attention to each movement your feet take, from the heels to the toes, from raising them off the ground to placing them back down. Walk slowly and deliberately, feeling the ground below you and the air around you. If you are outside, admire nature and take in all the sights, sounds, and smells you encounter.

5 When you return from your walking meditation, it will be time for another sitting meditation. For this practice, choose a meditation whose focus goes beyond your breath. For example, you might enjoy doing the Body Scan or Healing Self-Touch meditation at this time. Pick your favorite and relax into it.

6 If you feel hungry or thirsty after finishing your meditation, mindfully serve yourself a beverage or snack. If you are in the mood for a full meal, by all means enjoy one. If you are not hungry or thirsty, move on to either a movement or sitting meditation.

7 For movement, you could walk again or choose light stretching, some yoga, or Tai Chi. For a sitting meditation, you could go back to a simple breath meditation or select another meditation that calls to you at this time.

8 After this meditation, you can continue to alternate among sitting, walking, movement, and other meditations, interspersed with mindful eating, as your body requires, for as long as you like. Or, if you feel ready to conclude, you can use any (or all) of the following activities to bring your retreat to a close.

9 End your retreat by (1) journaling about your experience; (2) lighting a candle and saying a prayer; (3) drawing a bath and soaking in scented bubbles; and/or (4) lying in the yoga position known as Savasana (Corpse Pose).

10 When your retreat is over, mindfully rejoin the rest of your life. There is no need to rush back to your ordinary activities. Take your time. Partake in everyday mindfulness going forward. Allow the rewards from your retreat to linger.

MINDFUL BITE:

To center yourself and regain a posture of mindfulness when life around you gets challenging, meditate on this phrase:

Things are as they are. May I accept them as they are.

Conclusion

Drink your tea slowly and reverently, as if it is the axis on which the world earth revolves—slowly, evenly, without rushing toward the future; live the actual moment. Only this moment is life.

Thich Nhat Hanh

Here we are, at the end of the start of your journey to becoming a mindful eater. Congratulations on getting here. You have worked hard and by now, should be experiencing many of the benefits. Let's recap what you have accomplished.

In Step One, you began what I hope will be a lifelong meditation practice. You started small—only five minutes—and over time you built up your stamina so that you have or soon will reach the goal of thirty minutes most days. Because of your meditation practice, your mind is quieter, your focus and concentration have improved, and you are able to pause before automatically reacting to someone or something in your environment, including food.

Because of Step Two, you are in touch with your Inner Wisdom. You are tuned in to your body's signals for hunger, thirst, fullness, and satisfaction. You are making good choices about when and how much to feed your body.

As a result of Step Three, you are also making good choices about what to eat. You are balancing your eating selections with informative Outer Guidance. You now have a better understanding of the nutritional value of food and which foods serve you and your needs best. As a result, you may be seeing some of your excess weight starting to fall away.

Adding in Step Four allowed you to explore your emotions without overeating. Eating is no longer an automatic response to stress, anxiety, or other unpleasant emotions. You can now be with your emotions in a calm way and mindfully choose another way to deal with them.

Finally, with Step Five, you expanded mindfulness to the rest of your life. You now practice everyday mindfulness and derive more pleasure out of ordinary tasks. What a great place to be.

Moving forward, I would like to recommend you take these three steps:

(1) **Write down three things you can do to support your mindful eating practice.** Some examples include arranging a special place setting to celebrate your dining experience; inviting friends over for a mindful potluck dinner, guiding them through a mini meditation at the beginning of the meal; practicing the Raisin Exercise with different foods; increasing your meditation practice by either frequency or duration; and "riding the wave" of an emotion or craving to stop yourself from emotionally eating.

(2) **Identify any obstacles that may be getting in your way and make a plan to overcome them.** Review the section in Chapter Three which addresses Obstacles for guidance.

(3) **Review your meditation log and your journal.** If you have been keeping a meditation log and/or a journal, now is the time to revisit it. Seeing where you've been and how far you have come is encouraging. If you have not been keeping track in this way, start now. With an attitude of curiosity and non-judgement, make note of your challenges and your successes. Describe how your relationship with food has changed, how you have changed, and where you would like to go from here.

Remember Allison, whom I introduced to you in beginning of this journey? Here she is again as we come to the end of our work together.

After a few therapy sessions, Allison wanted to do the complete TAME Your Appetite program. She was uncomfortable doing it in a group, so we did the individual version. Over twelve sessions, Allison was taught what you were taught here: Mindfulness Meditation, Inner Wisdom, Outer Guidance, Handling Emotions, and Everyday Mindfulness.

At first, her weight did not change much, and she was disappointed, but, as we applied mindfulness to her weight loss goals, she was able to see weighing herself as a tool to assess what is working rather than an indictment of her efforts. Rather quickly, she became less interested in her weight and more interested in the impact mindfulness and mindful eating were having on her life. She described feeling "more at peace," "calmer," and "safer around food." She discovered that foods she previously coveted lost their appeal and new, more nutritious foods easily took their place. She felt "better in her own skin" and "more at ease with her husband and other family members." She slept better, coped with frustration with more ease, and above all, "liked who she became."

By the end of the twelve sessions, Allison had lost about twenty-five pounds, but what she found was more significant. She was "finally at peace with food." And for the first time ever "was convinced the weight would come off and stay off." Allison completed the full twelve session TAME Your Appetite program and then opted to join a continuity group. She continues to eat mindfully "more often than not," and is on her way to a healthy weight.

A FINAL WORD ABOUT SELF-COMPASSION

Before we end, I want to acknowledge that change is hard. As motivated as you may be to undo old eating habits and replace them with mindful ones, you will falter. We all do. If it were easy, you wouldn't need my help. To replace a lifetime of mindless and emotional eating with a new relationship to food and feelings takes time and perseverance. It also takes a healthy dose of self-compassion. I've mentioned self-compassion throughout this book. I'd like to conclude this part of our journey together with some instructions on how you can foster self-compassion as a tool to keep you moving forward to becoming a mindful eater and as a means for your personal growth. The self-compassion exercise I am about to share with you is adapted from the work of Kristen Neff, Ph.D., author of, *Self-Compassion: Stop Beating Yourself Up and Leave Insecurity Behind.*

Whenever you feel as if you are suffering or in distress of any kind, simply do this:

1   Place your hand(s) over your heart.

2   Take several slow deep breaths.

3   With a kind and gentle tone, repeat these phrases to yourself aloud or silently:

This is a moment of suffering.

Suffering is a part of life.

May I be kind to myself in this moment of suffering.

May I give myself the compassion I need at this time.

4   Remove your hand from your heart and go on with your day.

Practice Self-Compassion often. You cannot overdo it.

ON YOUR WAY...

What a wonderful journey we have been on. By adding a meditation practice to your life and cultivating Inner Wisdom and Outer Guidance, you have changed your relationships to food, yourself, and your life. You have learned to view your eating habits with openness and curiosity. Keep it going. Remember, through mindfulness training, you give up needing to control everything and come to accept reality as it is in each moment. With mindful awareness, you attend to yourself in the present, in the here and now. You experience the real, authentic you. You come to understand and appreciate your uniqueness. You arrive at a moment where you can make a different choice on how to respond to the circumstances you are facing. At first this can seem daunting, but with time and acceptance, it becomes a powerful tool for transformation. What a gift you have given yourself.

Celebrate yourself and your efforts. Keep doing what you are doing. Share what you have learned with others as you embrace mindful eating as your new way of life.

Until we meet again, I wish you peace with food and mindful habits.

—*Dr. Sheila*

Epilogue

A righteous man falls down seven times and gets up.

King Solomon, Proverbs, 24:16

Wednesday, April 15, 2020, was the worst day of my life. On that day, my beloved mother died from COVID-19. She was eighty-nine years old, living in a Senior Community in Westchester County, New York (the epicenter of the pandemic at that moment) when she fell ill. She was hospitalized and in a matter of days, she was gone.

Because she was in New York and I was in Los Angeles, I could not attend her funeral. My sister, other family members and friends were able to be graveside as the Rabbi held up an iPad so I could watch. I gave my mother's eulogy over Zoom. We also held Shiva (the Jewish mourning tradition) via Zoom. There I was in my makeshift home office grieving my mother online.

The distance and isolation the pandemic caused left me broken. I reached out to my support system for help, and they rallied. But it was hard. I managed to show up for my patients, clients, and students on a regular basis, but when I was not working, I was grieving.

Understanding the nature of grief, I gave myself permission to feel whatever I felt and to do whatever I needed to do to take care of myself. Some days that meant eating mindfully, practicing meditation, exercising, and journaling. Other days, it meant eating cereal from the box and watching reruns of *Schitt's Creek* for hours.

Many of my mindful healthy habits slipped away as I grappled with my loss. I was okay with that because I knew that I could always begin again. And I did, on and off for months.

Because of the length and breadth of the pandemic, I was unable to get to New York until the end of July 2021. For three days I was with my New York family and friends. For three days we laughed and cried over mom. Finally, on the last day, we went to her grave for a small service, and I got to say goodbye in person.

Upon my return to Los Angeles, I felt a weight lift off my shoulders. It took a little while longer, but on August 15, 2021, exactly sixteen months from the day I lost my mother, I began again.

My daily meditation practice returned. My mindful eating habits reemerged. I walked every day and slept through the night. The weight I gained (which was more in line with an American Psychological Association's study which said Americans gained an average of twenty-nine pounds, not fifteen pounds, during the pandemic) started to come off.

I am sharing this with you to let you know, even though I am an "expert," I am not perfect. Life happens. Death happens. Mindlessness happens. Mindfulness happens.

I know I was not the only person who suffered greatly as a result of the pandemic. If you suffered too, you have my deepest sympathies. If during the pandemic you were not at your finest, if your habits and healthy efforts fell by the wayside, it's okay. No judgement. Just begin again.

My hope is that this book will help you do just that—begin again.

Additional Resources

APPS

Calm

Headspace

Insight Timer

BOOKS

Books by Dr. Sheila

Do You Use Food to Cope? A Comprehensive 15-Week Program for Overcoming Emotional Overeating, published by Writer's Club Press, 2002.

Manage Your Emotions, Manage Your Weight, (eBook), available at the store on TAMEYourAppetite.com.

Self-Fullness: The Art of Loving and Caring for Your 'Self,' published by Writer's Club Press, 2000.

Stop Dieting, Start Living, (eBook), available at the store on www.TAMEYourAppetite.com.

The Best Diet Begins in Your Mind, Eliminate the Eight Emotional Obstacles to Permanent Weight Loss, published by iUniverse, 2015.

Books on Meditation

Mindfulness Meditation for Beginners, by J. Kabat-Zinn.
Real Happiness, by Sharon Salzberg, published by Workman Publishing, 2011.
Soul-Centered, by Sarah McLean, published by Hay House, Inc., 2012.

Books on Mindful Eating

Mindful Eating, by Jan Chazen Bays, M.D., published by Shambhala, 2009.

Mindful Emotional Eating, by Pavel G. Somov, Ph.D., published by PESI Publishing & Media, 2015.

Nourishing Wisdom, by David Marc, published by Bell Tower Books, 1992.

The Mindful Diet, by Ruth Wolever, Ph.D. and Beth Reardon, published by Scribner, 2015.

The Joy of Half a Cookie, by Jena Kristeller, Ph.D., published by Penguin, 2015.

The Zen of Eating, by Ronna Kabatznick, Ph.D., published by Pedigree, 1998.

Well Nourished, by Andrea Lieberstein, MPH, RDN, published by Fair Winds Press, 2017.

Books on Mindfulness

A Path with Heart, by Jack Kornfield, published by Bantam, 1993.

Coming to Our Senses: Healing Ourselves and the World through Mindfulness, by J. Kabat-Zinn, published by Hyperion, 2006.

Full Catastrophe Living, by J. Kabat-Zinn.

Fully Present, by Susan Smalley and Diana Winston, published by First Da Capo Press, 2010.

Mindfulness in Plain English, by H. Gunaratana, published by Wisdom Publications, 1991.

Self-Compassion: Stop Beating Yourself Up and Leave Your Insecurities Behind, by Kristen Neff, Ph.D., published by William Morrow, 2011.

The Miracle of Mindfulness, by Thich Nat Hanh.

Touching Peace, by Thich Nat Hanh.

True Refuge: Finding Peace and Freedom in Your Own Awakened Heart, by Tara Brach, published by Random House, 2013.

Wherever You Are, There You Are, by J. Kabat-Zinn.

You Are Not Your Pain, by Vidyamala Burch and Danny Penman.

Books Mentioned

8 Weeks to Optimum Health, by Andrew Weil, M.D.

Eat to Live, by Joel Furhman, M.D.

Fully Present: The Science, Art, and Practice of Mindfulness, by Susan Smalley and Diana Winston

Macular Degeneration: The Complete Guide to Saving and Maximizing Your Sight, by Lylas Mogk, MD.

Mindfulness-Based Therapy for Insomnia, by Jason C. Ong, Ph.D.

Never Be Sick Again, by Raymond Francis, M.Sc.

The Artist's Way, by Julia Cameron

The Eat-Clean Diet, by Tosca Reno, B.Sc.

WEBSITES

Chopracentermeditations.com

HayHouse.com

marc.ucla.edu

SoundsTrue.com

TAMEYourAppetite.com

TheCenterForMindfulEating.org (TCME.org)

Research References

Alberts, Mulkens, Smeets, and Thewissen, *Coping with Food Cravings, Appetite*. 55(1) 160–163 (2010).

Chiesa, Serretti, Mindfulness-Based Stress Reduction for Stress Management in Healthy People, *Journal of Alternative and Complementary Medicine* 15(5) 593–600.

Daubenmier, Kristeller, Hecht et al., Mindfulness Intervention for Stress Eating to Reduce Cortisol and Abdominal Fat among Overweight and Obese Women: An Exploratory Randomized Controlled Study, *Journal of Obesity*, (2011): doi: 1155/2011/651936.

Fothergill et al., *Obesity*, 24: 1612–19 (2016).

Kristeller et al., *Mindfulness*, 5: 282–297 (2014).

Kristeller and Wolever, Mindfulness-Based Eating Awareness Training for Treating Binge Eating Disorder: The Conceptual Foundation, *Eating Disorders*, 19: 1, 49–61 (2011).

Kristeller, Wolever, and Sheets, Mindfulness-Based Eating Awareness Training (MB-EAT) for Binge Eating Disorder: A Randomized Clinical Trial, *Mindfulness* 3, no. 4 (2012): doi: 10.1007/s1267-012-0179-1.

Leong, Madden Gray, Water and Howath, Faster Self-Reported Speed of Eating is Related to Higher Body Mass Index in a Nationwide Survey of Middle-Aged Women, *Journal of American Dietetic Association* 111: 1192-97,doi:10.106/j.jada2011.05.012.

Mason, Epel, Aschbacher, Lustig, Acree, and Kristeller, SHINE Randomized Controlled Trial, *Appetite*, 100, 86–93 (2016).

Sumithran & Proietto, *Clinical Science*, 124:231–41 (2013).

Wansink and Sobal, Mindless Eating: The 200 Daily Food Decisions We Overlook, *Environment and Behavior*, 39 (1)106–23.

Weir, Kirsten. The Extra Weight of COVID-19. American Psychological Association, July 2021. https://www.apa.org/monitor/2021/07/extra-weight-covid.

An Exploratory Study of a Meditation-based Intervention for Binge Eating Disorder. *Journal of Health Psychology*, Vol 4(3) 357–363: 008561 (1999).

Comparative Effectiveness of a Mindful Eating Intervention to a Diabetes Self-Management Intervention among Adults with Type 2 Diabetes: A Pilot Study *Journal of the Academy of Nutrition and Dietetics* (2012).

Comparison of a Mindful Eating Intervention to a Diabetes Self-Management Intervention Among Adults with Type 2 Diabetes: A Randomized Controlled *Trial Health Education & Behavior* Vol. 41(2) 145–154 (2014).

Eating Quickly and Until Full Triples Risk of Being Overweight, *ScienceDaily* 2008/10/081021210307 (2008).

https://www.apa.org/monitor/2021/07/extra-weight-covid

Join our Community

Become part of Dr. Sheila's mindful eating community by joining:

Newsletter: TAMEYourAppetite.com
Facebook: facebook.com/TAMEAppetite/
Twitter: @TAMEAppetite
LinkedIn: linkedin.com/in/drsheila/
Instagram: @tameappetite/

About the Author

Dr. Sheila Forman holds a Ph.D. in Psychology and practiced psychotherapy for over twenty years before becoming a Mindfulness-Based Eating Awareness Training (MB-EAT) Instructor. For her entire career, Dr. Sheila has been helping people address weight and food issues by teaching how to cope with emotions without overeating and, more recently, how to eliminate mindless eating with mindfulness meditation and other mindful skills and techniques.

Her program, *TAME Your Appetite – The Art of Mindful Eating,* is a non-diet approach to weight management, incorporating all that Dr. Sheila knows about healing emotional and mindless eating.

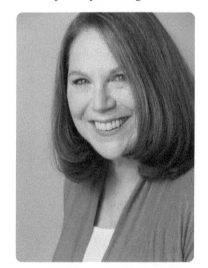

For more information about *TAME*, go to TAMEYourAppetite.com or email Dr. Sheila at Info@TAMEYourAppetite.com.

Published by

TVGUESTPERT PUBLISHING

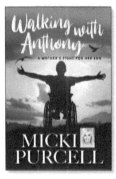

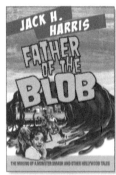

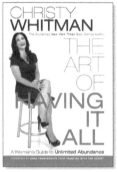

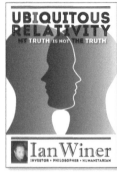

MICKI PURCELL
Walking With Anthony:
A Mother's Fight For Her
Son
Hardcover $22.95
Kindle: $9.99

JACK H. HARRIS
Father of the Blob:
The Making of a Monster
Smash and Other
Hollywood Tales
Paperback: $16.95
Kindle/Nook: $9.99

New York Times Best Seller
CHRISTY WHITMAN
The Art of Having It
All: A Woman's Guide to
Unlimited Abundance
Paperback: $16.95
Kindle/Nook: $9.99
Audible Book: $13.00

IAN WINER
Ubiquitous Relativity: My
Truth is Not the Truth
Paperback: $16.95
Kindle: $9.99

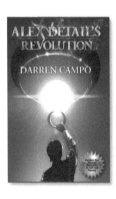

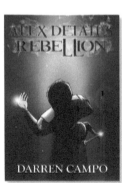

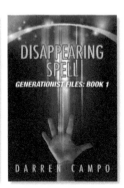

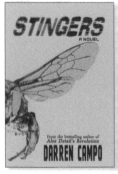

DARREN CAMPO
Alex Detail's Revolution
Paperback: $9.95
Hardcover: $22.95
Kindle: $9.15

DARREN CAMPO
Alex Detail's Rebellion
Hardcover: $22.95
Kindle: $9.99

DARREN CAMPO
Disappearing Spell:
Generationist Files:
Book 1
Kindle: $2.99

DARREN CAMPO
Stingers
Paperback: $9.99
Kindle: $9.99

TVGuestpert Publishing
11664 National Blvd, #345
Los Angeles, CA. 90064
310-584-1504
www.TVGPublishing.com

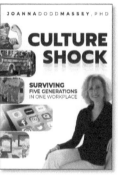 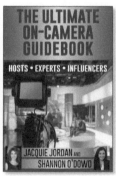 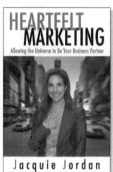 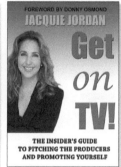

JOANNA DODD
MASSEY
*Culture Shock: Surviving
Five Generations in One
Workplace*
Paperback: $16.95
Kindle/Nook: $9.99

JACQUIE JORDAN AND
SHANNON O'DOWD
*The Ultimate On-
Camera Guidebook:
Hosts*Experts*Influencers*
Paperback: $16.95
Kindle: $9.99

JACQUIE JORDAN
*Heartfelt Marketing:
Allowing the Universe to Be
Your Business Partner*
Paperback: $15.95
Kindle: $9.99
Audible: $9.95

JACQUIE JORDAN
*Get on TV! The Insider's
Guide to Pitching the
Producers and Promoting
Yourself*
Published by Sourcebooks
Paperback: $14.95
Kindle: $9.99
Nook: $14.95

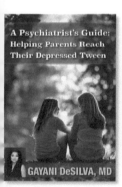 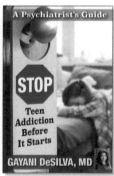 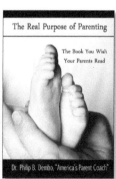 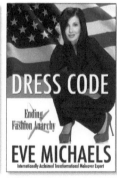

GAYANI DESILVA, MD
*A Psychiatrist's Guide: Helping
Parents Reach Their Depressed
Tween*
Paperback: $16.95
Kindle: $9.99

GAYANI DESILVA, MD
*A Psychiatrist's Guide: Stop
Teen Addiction Before It
Starts*
Paperback: $16.95
Kindle: $9.99
Audible: $14.95

DR. PHILIP DEMBO
*The Real Purpose of
Parenting: The Book You
Wish Your Parents Read*
Paperback: $15.95
Kindle: $9.99
Audible: $23.95

EVE MICHAELS
*Dress Code: Ending
Fashion Anarchy*
Paperback: $15.95
Kindle/Nook: $9.99
Audible Book: $17.95

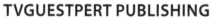

Published by
TVGUESTPERT PUBLISHING

TVGuestpert Publishing
11664 National Blvd, #345
Los Angeles, CA. 90064
310-584-1504
www.TVGPublishing.com

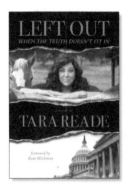

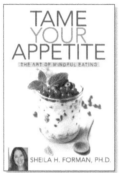

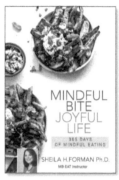

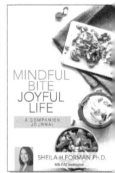

TARA READE
Left Out: When The Truth Doesn't Fit In
Hardcover: $22.95
Kindle: $9.99

SHEILA H. FORMAN, Ph.D
Tame Your Appetite: The Art of Mindful Eating
Paperback: $16.95
Kindle: $9.99

SHEILA H. FORMAN, Ph.D
Mindful Bite Joyful Life; 365 Days of Mindful Eating
*Coming Soon

SHEILA H. FORMAN, Ph.D
Mindful Bite Joyful Life; A Companion Journal
*Coming Soon